Praise for *Keto Flex*

"Ben Azadi has been a great resource to the low-carb and fasting community. Ben's new book, Keto Flex, *explores different applications of ways to diet and fasting, because there's not a one-size-fits-all approach when it comes to your health.* Keto Flex *provides the latest in research and practical strategies. This is a great read for understanding weight loss, health, and longevity."*

—**Dr. Jason Fung,** *New York Times* best-selling author of *The Obesity Code*

"We all want to be healthy and lean. And while there is no single variable that dictates metabolic health, the best evidence shows that the food we eat matters most. This is where Ben Azadi comes in. In Keto Flex, *Ben lays out a strategy for drastically improving metabolic health with simple steps that involve adjusting not only what you eat, but also when you eat. If you're searching for a clearer view of your health, this book will provide the insight and strategy you've been looking for."*

—**Dr. Benjamin Bikman**, author of *Why We Get Sick*

"Ben is one of the most trusted sources in the ketogenic community, and Keto Flex *simply makes sense. Our bodies have the ability to know how to regulate body fat; if we can just allow the ketogenic diet to do its part while letting the body do its part, we can live a flexible, nonrestrictive lifestyle that gets our bodies and our emotions what they want! Go Ben! What a great book!"*

—**Thomas A. DeLauer**, author, health expert, and performance coach

"Ben Azadi is not only one of the smartest guys in the industry, but he's also a genius at breaking things down for people so that literally everyone can understand the step-by-step protocols he's put together to help others achieve optimal health. His book Keto Flex *does just that! A super-simple 4-step process that can't go wrong!"*

—**Drew Manning,** *New York Times* best-selling author of *Fit2Fat2Fit*

"In easy-to-follow, simple steps and rules, Ben Azadi provides you with a clear blueprint for everyone to take control of their waistline, blood sugar, and other metabolic markers. These time-tested methods are simple, practical ways to regain control of your health using natural dietary methods instead of medications."

—**Megan Ramos**, clinical researcher, author of *Life in the Fasting Lane*

"Ben Azadi is, without a doubt, one of the emerging leaders in the keto, low-carb space. His knowledge, enthusiasm, and positivity are infectious, and his take on ketogenic diets is refreshing. I love that Ben's approach takes into account bio-individuality and fully embraces finding your own path to wellness."

—**Cynthia Thurlow**, nurse practitioner, women's health expert

"Ben is the most passionate and experienced keto guru! His new book, Keto Flex, *is a fantastic read for anyone interested in the keto diet! From the beginner to the experienced keto dieter, this book has the tips that will help you succeed!"*

—**Maria Emmerich**, best-selling author of *The Carnivore Cookbook* and *Keto Comfort Foods*

"Ben Azadi is a daring soldier in the decades-long war against dietary lies that turn well-meaning doctors into unwitting agents of disease. Ben's track record of pulling casualties from the field and bringing them back to health should earn him some kind of nutritional Purple Heart. We need more strong voices like Ben's, and we need more books like Ben's Keto Flex.*"*

—**Cate Shanahan, MD,** *New York Times* best-selling author of *The Fatburn Fix, Deep Nutrition,* and *Dark Calories*

"Ben has come out with a great book about doing a sustainable ketogenic diet. Too often do authors and dieticians fall into the trap of their own dogma, but Keto Flex *circumvents that. Ben hits the nail on the head by implementing the concept of metabolic flexibility that allows the person to achieve optimal fat-burning and glucose tolerance. I think every person should go through some periods of keto-adaptation to prime their body for burning fat and ketones. However, it isn't necessary to stay in ketosis for the rest of your life to maintain those benefits. The steps outlined by Ben will help the person reach that state with ease and less stress. Besides the book, Ben is also working hard in inspiring people and helping them to transform their health."*

—**Siim Land**, author of *Metabolic Autophagy*

"Focusing on the balance of Fasting and Feasting is a powerful and ancestrally-informed strategy for transformation, vibrant health, and longevity. Since there is no magic bullet or one-size-fits-all approach, flexibility is critical to get results that last. We need Ben's insight and voice more than ever!"

—**Abel James,** *New York Times* best-selling author and creator of *Fat-Burning Man*

"Ben has a unique way of taking a scientific approach yet breaking it down into easy, understandable, and most importantly, practical steps for you to apply on your keto journey. Keto Flex *provides the latest science and applications for the ketogenic lifestyle with practical tips on how you can get started today. This is a must-read for anyone looking to optimize their body and brain through ketogenic nutrition with practical advice on how to get started and sustain this lifestyle for years to come!"*

—**Ryan Lowery,** co-author of *The Ketogenic Bible*

"I am so thrilled Ben wrote this book! No one is more tenacious and thoughtful at empowering people to step into their greatness. In the ketogenic world, there has been a massive hole in information providing people the tools to properly move in and out of ketosis. Not only does Ben fill that hole with this book, but he eloquently lays out foundational principles of the ketogenic diet that so many are missing. This book is a game changer for anyone wanting to build a ketogenic lifestyle!"

—**Dr. Mindy Pelz,** best-selling author of *Fast Like a Girl*

"Ben Azadi is one of the top thought leaders in the space of keto and intermittent fasting. His new book, Keto Flex, brings together the benefits of a low-carb lifestyle, intermittent fasting, nutrient timing, and carb cycling for optimal energy, fat-burning, and hormone balance. I highly recommend this book to anyone who wants to improve their brain and body!

—**Dr. David Jockers, DNM, DC, MS,** author of *Keto Metabolic Breakthrough* and *The Fasting Transformation*

KETO FLEX

REVISED

ALSO BY BEN AZADI

Metabolic Freedom: A 30-Day Guide to Restore Your Metabolism, Heal Hormones & Burn Fat

All of the above are available at your local bookstore, or may be ordered by visiting:

Hay House USA: www.hayhouse.com®
Hay House Australia: www.hayhouse.com.au
Hay House UK: www.hayhouse.co.uk
Hay House India: www.hayhouse.co.in

KETO FLEX

REVISED

THE ADVANCED GUIDE TO METABOLIC FLEXIBILITY, FAT BURNING, AND HORMONE HEALTH FOR EVERY BODY AT EVERY STAGE

BEN AZADI

HAY HOUSE

HAY HOUSE LLC
Carlsbad, California • New York City
London • Sydney • New Delhi

Published in the United States by: Hay House LLC, www.hayhouse.com®
P.O. Box 5100, Carlsbad, CA, 92018-5100

Indexer: J S Editorial, LLC
Cover design: Christopher Tobias
Interior design: Nick C. Welch

Tradepaper ISBN: 979-8-3186-0252-8
E-book ISBN: 979-8-3186-0253-5
Audiobook ISBN: 979-8-3186-0254-2

2nd Printing

Printed in the United States of America

I want to dedicate this book to two amazing women in my life: my mother, Haddi Azadi, and my wife, Natassia Coelho. Mom, thank you for the tremendous support you continue to provide. You're the most unselfish person I've ever met in my life. I am living the American dream because of the sacrifices you and Dad made. I love you. Natassia, your support and love for me is daily oxygen for my soul. I love you.

I also want to dedicate this book to Keto Kampers all over the world. I call you the 3 percenters because you think differently than most of the world. While others chase symptoms, I applaud you for searching for the root cause.

CONTENTS

FOREWORD

This book offers a genuine solution for individuals dealing with challenges in weight loss, encountering plateaus, experiencing low energy and brain fog, or seeking to enhance their overall health.

Many years ago, my wife and I both started a keto diet. Within days, my ketones were soaring, and I felt amazing. The first thing I noticed was that my brain clicked on, and I could recall facts and figures like never before. I felt like Superman with boundless energy! I even gained muscle and lost fat. In contrast, my wife, Merily, did not experience the same success. Her ketone levels were barely getting over .4 to .5 (.8 to 1.8 is a good average for being in keto), and she was anything but thriving. I advised her to lower her carbs even more. That didn't work. Her energy declined and her ketones didn't move. I suggested that it might take her more time to adapt.

After a few months, it became clear this was not the case. Out of frustration and having no answers, I advised Merily to go back to a higher-carb, healthy diet. She did—and felt better right away. After a month or two, I suggested she give keto another try, and this time her ketones were a little better, and so too was her energy. That's when I came up with the idea to move her out of ketosis again for another month and move her back in once again. The third time, it worked. She was thriving, and her ketones were over 1.0 consistently.

After this experience, I decided to try this carbohydrate-cycling approach with some patients who had been struggling in keto or just with weight-loss resistance in general. It worked! Then I took the idea to my practitioners and doctors I coached and asked them to try this "diet variation" concept, and the results were the same. Diet variation was born. There are monthly and weekly strategies that work amazingly well for individuals who have challenges with thyroid, adrenal, and low hormones. The variation forces the body to adapt to the change, and it adapts by optimizing hormones.

Being one of my students, Ben took this concept and made it easy and usable for people to put into practice, as Ben does with most things. *Keto Flex* was born. This book is a user-friendly guide to a new concept in the low-carb awakening that is sweeping the planet.

As it turns out, the concept is based on solid science. When you change your diet, even adding weekly feast days and famine days, the body must adapt to the abrupt changes, which leads to hormone optimization. Hormones are at the heart of why people stop losing weight, can't lose weight, or don't have success on a healthy diet when others do.

Recently I had the pleasure of interviewing Krista Varady, PhD, a professor of nutrition at the University of Illinois, Chicago. She discussed her study on what she called "alternate-day dieting." Her study compared many different diets with the concept of eating the standard American diet one day and then a diet of very restricted calories the next (feast/famine). The feast/famine worked better than all the other diets for weight loss. I asked why she thought this was the case, and she said, "It's all about adaptation."

How does the body adapt? It optimizes our hormones, and the benefit is that we become more efficient fat burners. It's all about using the body's natural survival mechanisms. The number-one priority of the body is always survival. I have studied very healthy ancient cultures and have found that they were invariably forced into diet changes, and therefore I believe we are programmed for this. Our bad genes that get triggered by the stressors that lead to disease get turned off. Our microbiome (gut bacteria), which is responsible for 70 percent of our immune system, resets and becomes more diverse. All this leads to better health.

Keto Flex will teach you how to add this incredible concept to your daily life. Ben makes it so easy, and I predict you will not only experience an amazing breakthrough, but also you will find that it is easier for you to stay on a healthy diet.

You are blessed to have this book in your hands.

—Dr. Daniel Pompa, drpompa.com,
leading expert on cellular health

INTRODUCTION

This book can transform your life. Well, to a point. It can't make you rich or turn you into a celebrity—you'll have to get those on your own. But it can do something just as valuable. Perhaps even *more* valuable. It can offer a beacon of hope, a road map to guide you back to wellness and vitality.

I recognize firsthand the struggles you face daily: the relentless battle against brain fog, the persistent grip of chronic fatigue, and the frustrating weight-loss resistance. Perhaps you're grappling with the challenges of diabetes and high blood sugar levels or the burden of autoimmune conditions weighing heavily upon you. Maybe you're encountering insulin resistance, digestive woes, or soaring blood pressure. These symptoms, though formidable adversaries, are not insurmountable obstacles—they are opportunities for transformation. I once had many of these symptoms too: knee pain, lower-back pain, prediabetes, chronic fatigue, inflammation, and more. And I was 80 pounds overweight. Until I found my way back to health by consuming the right foods, flexing in and out of ketosis, and practicing the ancient tool of intermittent fasting (IF).

Whether you're 20 years old or 90 years old, *Keto Flex* will change the way you view health. As we explore the interference that has led to your symptoms and work on removing them one by one, you'll get your life back and feel better than ever.

WHAT IS KETO FLEX?

How would you like to wake up in the morning without an alarm clock, full of energy? This energy lasts throughout the entire day without any dips, even after eating. It doesn't rely on coffee or a midafternoon sugar rush. In fact, you don't have to do a darn thing other than *eat*.

Crazy, right?

Of course, it all depends on *what* you eat and *when* you eat it.

I'll show you how the familiar mix of everyday nutrients—protein, fat, and carbohydrates—can change, making a big difference in your health. You'll see how cutting carbs and consuming more fat and protein will change the way your body creates the energy it needs to live and thrive.

I can hear brakes screeching.

"Stop!" you say. "You want me to eat *more fat*?"

Yes.

Healthy fats have been maligned by the processed-foods industry because it wants you to consume sugar, corn syrup, and artificial sweeteners, which *really are* bad for you. Healthy fats, such as found in olive oil, avocados, eggs, butter, beef, and much more, provide the nutrition you need and fill you up while allowing your body to shift from burning glucose—a sugar—to making ketones, which can also be used for energy. Your body makes ketones from the fat cells you already have. These fat cells are nature's ancient source of free energy for your body. They are waiting to be accessed, which happens when certain conditions are met. Burning fat will rehab your cells and keep your hormones performing at their best, improving your health, your symptoms, and your waistline. In this book you'll find helpful lists of which foods to avoid and which foods to include.

The key is not only *what* you eat but also *when* you eat. Thousands of years ago, our ancestors were accustomed to having sporadic supplies of food. They didn't always eat three meals a day. To them this was normal, and the human digestive system was designed to function optimally with long periods between meals. Fasting helps our body eliminate toxins and can have a positive effect on cardiometabolic, digestive, and brain health. I'll teach you how to replicate those ancient conditions—which your digestive system will embrace—with deliberate, intermittent fasting. This dietary "flex" kickstarts the process of ketone production and puts you on the road to shedding excess fat, feeling good about yourself, and enjoying better health.

What sets the Keto Flex Reset apart is that it takes into account our primal brain's instincts for survival—it eases us into ketosis gradually, ensures that the food we're eating keeps us full, and gives us "feast days," where we decrease our fasting time and increase carbs. This reassures our brain that we're not going to starve. The Keto Flex Reset includes four pillars:

1. Adapt: gradually transitioning from burning sugar to burning fat
2. Fast: incorporating intermittent-fasting strategies to accelerate fat burning and healing
3. Phase: practicing the carnivore diet to phase out all antinutrients
4. Flex: flexing in and out of ketosis

The flex piece is important, because we want our body to achieve metabolic flexibility and easily move between fat burning and sugar burning. It's all about teaching our body to adapt to change, which strengthens our good cells and eliminates our weak ones. I introduced this concept in my book *Metabolic Freedom*, and *Keto Flex* now offers a more advanced, customized version of the Metabolic Freedom Reset. I've also incorporated additional information on how to follow this program if you're diabetic (one of my personal goals is to help as many people as possible reverse their type 2 diabetes). And I've included a special chapter for women on how to coordinate the reset with their cycle or adjust it if they are postmenopausal. Finally, I address some of the most common symptoms that may occur—from sugar cravings to sleep issues—and offer my time-tested solutions. To make your Keto Flex lifestyle supereasy, this book includes delicious fat-burning meal plans, recipes, and shopping lists.

GET READY FOR REMARKABLE RESULTS!

I've applied the principles in this book to thousands of my Fat Loss Academy students, and the results have been nothing short of incredible. I've seen type 2 insulin-dependent students who have been taking insulin for more than 10 years apply these principles and work with their doctors to completely wean off insulin. I've seen weight-loss resistance become a thing of the past. And I've even seen people with stage 4 cancer who have been given months to live go on to heal themselves. And all thanks to the Keto Flex lifestyle.

Owen Hemsath discovered Keto Flex after he'd been diagnosed with stage 4 metastatic cancer. He'd already survived stage 3 thymoma, a cancer of the thymus gland, in 2015 and endured a year of aggressive chemotherapy followed by the highest legal amount of radiation. His body was never the same again. Feeling broken and battered, he spent the next few years riddled with side effects and a constant fear of recurrence. In 2020 his body gave out and his wife rushed him to the hospital, where they received the devastating news that his cancer had returned—more powerful than ever. It had overwhelmed his body and was unresponsive to chemo. The doctors gave him two years to live.

He found one of my interviews about the benefits of fasting for cancer patients and decided to try keto flexing. Owen emptied his cabinets of flour, sugar, and processed crackers and cookies and replaced them with whole foods, clean meats, and lots of grass-fed butter. Within three weeks of eating keto, his side effects were gone, and within three months he'd lost 50 pounds and was feeling healthier than ever. He was back in the gym, lifting weights and running a few miles per week, and had to buy all new clothes.

While skeptical, his oncologist suggested a follow-up CT scan to see where his cancer had progressed. Owen was shocked when he received the test results: His tumors had shrunk by 30 percent! As he continued his ketogenic diet, his tumors continued to shrink, and his health continued to improve. It became his primary strategy for healing his cancer, and in spring 2022, his scans showed that he was now cancer-free. Even though he'd been given only two years to live, in just one and a half years, there was no detectable cancer in his body.

Now Owen is five years beyond his stage 4 diagnosis and healthier than ever. He continues to practice keto and fasting and is so grateful to spend more time with his wife and kids. He's not a cancer survivor . . . but a cancer thriver. For a deeper dive into Owen's journey, I interviewed him on the *Metabolic Freedom* podcast (Episode 407), where he shared his full story in his own words.

Whether you have a life-threatening disease like Owen, an autoimmune disorder, diabetes, fatigue, or a host of other uncomfortable symptoms, the Keto Flex lifestyle can help you feel better. Just stay focused on the positive outcome, and before you know it, you'll start to notice those pesky symptoms subsiding, the weight-loss resistance disappearing, and your energy, concentration, and health returning.

Ready to transform your life? Let's get started!

CHAPTER ONE

CELLULAR REHAB

Your body is built of cells. Trillions of them.[1] Why am I including a chapter on cells in a book about keto? Because your overall health *begins* in your cells. Unhealthy cells lead to brain fog, fatigue, weight-loss resistance, obesity, digestive issues, and many other symptoms you may be experiencing. We need to rehabilitate our cells, and the Keto Flex Reset does just that.

In this chapter I'll introduce the parts of our cells and the crucial relationship between DNA and RNA when it comes to creating healthier ones. I'll explain how the mitochondria within our cells convert food into energy, where that energy comes from—sugar and fat—and which one is better (hint: It's not the sweet one). We'll also explore the various hormones that affect our cells, specifically those tied to our weight regulation, how our toxic environment can disrupt hormone function, and what we can do about it.

THE PARTS OF OUR CELLS (AND THEIR IMPORTANT ROLES)

There are many different types of cells with individual functions, but every cell consists of three basic parts: the cell membrane, the nucleus, and—between the two—the cytoplasm. The cell membrane functions as the outer "skin" of the cell, controlling the passage of materials into and out of the cell. It's composed of a double layer of phospholipid molecules. (*Lipid* means "fatty." Yep, there's that word again!) Proteins in the cell membrane provide various services, including structural support and the formation of channels for the passage of materials. The cell membrane's job is to protect the cell, allowing in the nutrients it needs while guarding against harmful substances like toxins and viruses.

The nucleus is the control center of the cell. It determines how the cell will function, as well as the basic structure of the cell. It contains our DNA and RNA. Our DNA is like a handbook stored inside our cells—it contains all the genetic instructions passed down from our parents. We can't change the DNA we were given at birth. What we can change is the *expression* of our genes, which is called epigenetics. We can train our body to read the parts of the DNA that create healthy cells, tissues, skin, organs, and so on, and we can turn off the bad instructions. This means that you actually have some control over those symptoms you've been experiencing.

RNA is the messenger to help this epigenetics process—it's the method by which the body acts out the instructions. The problem is that when our cells become inflamed and/or nutrient deficient, DNA and RNA communication breaks down. This is what makes keto flexing so empowering—when you learn how to fuel your body with the right ingredients, you reduce that inflammation, reestablish that communication, and express the genes that lead to better health.

Our internal and external environments affect our cells. Inflammatory foods and environmental toxins injure our DNA, and we must repair it several times a day. According to the research of Dr. Zach Bush, an internationally recognized educator and thought leader on the microbiome as it relates to health, disease, and food systems, in just seconds the micro-RNA can adapt. A single gene can make more than 200 different proteins. Who decides which genes are made? The micro-RNA. With our 20,000 genes, we can build four million different variants of ourselves. When we're diagnosed with cancer or heart disease, we're told that this disease was "in our genes" or just bad luck. But that's not entirely true, because we hold the key to determining which genes get expressed and which ones don't. About 5 percent of the miRNA in our blood right now is from the food we eat (meat and plants), 15 percent is from the bacteria in our environment (the genus *Escherichia*, best known for *E. coli*, originates in the intestinal tracts of humans and animals, yet its genetic fingerprints can be found throughout our environment—in soil, water, plants, and food), and 15 percent is from the fungi in our environment. Some fungi, like mushrooms, are beneficial and help us absorb nutrients, while others, like certain molds, are parasitic and cause us harm.

We are what we eat. We are also the *stress* of what we eat. If you have a conventional cow raised on a feeding lot, the stress of the cow will be transferred to the health of the human being who consumes it. Scientists believe this is happening mostly through our micro-RNA.

The cytoplasm is the gelatinous fluid that fills the cell. It provides support for the hundreds of organelles, which are the subcellular structures with specific jobs to perform in the cell, much like the organs in the body. All the functions for cell expansion, growth, and replication are carried out in the cytoplasm of a cell. By switching cells to fat and ketones, fasting and ketogenic nutrition reprogram the cytoplasm—dialing down mTOR (a protein kinase that contributes to various diseases), nudging up autophagy (the removal of damaged cells), and strengthening redox defenses (which protect against oxidative stress)—effects shown in human studies of time-restricted eating, short fasts, and nutritional ketosis.

THE LIFESPAN OF A CELL

Most of the cells in your body die and are replaced by identical copies regularly through a process called *apoptosis*. Your body doesn't leave you hanging; it creates a new cell via stem cells to replace the dead cell. You are literally not the same person you were a few years ago. You look the same and may behave the same, but your actual cells are different.

Here's a good analogy. You may have heard of the USS *Constitution*, fondly called "Old Ironsides." This wooden warship was launched in 1797 and finally retired from active service in 1881. She's still a commissioned Navy vessel—the oldest ship to have that designation. At her berth in the old Charlestown Navy Yard in Boston, she's well cared for. As the decades have passed, the wooden parts have rotted, and the metal parts have rusted or corroded. Periodically, the ship is dry-docked, and the damaged parts are replaced with identical new parts. This has been done so often that the ship is now estimated to be 85 percent replaced. Only 15 percent—mainly the massive keel of white oak—is original. Yet if a sailor from the 19th century were to be magically transported to the ship today, he'd be hard-pressed to see the changes. For all practical purposes, Old Ironsides is the same ship she was back in 1797. Your body is repaired and replaced in much the same way. In an adult, each day as many as 100 billion cells die and are replaced by other cells.

This process of natural cell renewal is called *programmed cell death*. It plays a key role in balancing cell proliferation and maintaining constant cell numbers in the tissues as well as being one of the first lines of defense against cancer and infection by invaders such as viruses.

You may be wondering about fat cells. Your body can make new ones, and the number of fat cells increases through childhood and adolescence and then generally stabilizes in adulthood.

However, fat cells can change in size. Unlike most other types of cells, which cannot change their size, fat cells will expand and contract with weight gain or weight loss. And like most cell types in the body, they eventually die and are replaced by new fat cells. Cell death and new cell production appear to be tightly coupled. About 10 percent of fat cells die each year and are replaced at the same rate.

Beyond their role in storing fat, fat cells secrete hormones and proteins that affect energy metabolism. Some scientists believe that while *losing* weight is relatively easy, it may be hard to *keep it off* because as fat cells become smaller, they may send signals to increase appetite and fat storage.

To survive and thrive, every cell in your body must have a constant supply of vital substances such as glucose, oxygen, and trace minerals, and it must be able to dispose of waste products, including lactic acid, acetic acid, carbon dioxide, ammonia, and urea. Before we discuss the best strategies for maintaining optimal cell health, we need to learn about glucose, glycogen, and ketones.

HOW WE GET ENERGY: GLUCOSE VS. KETONES

If you study how the body transforms various molecules into energy, you'll learn about the Krebs cycle. It's a series of chemical reactions used to release stored energy through the oxidation of acetyl coenzyme A (acetyl-CoA) derived from carbohydrates, fats, and proteins. The cycle also provides precursors of certain amino acids, as well as the reducing agent NADH, which are used in numerous other reactions. It's named after Hans A. Krebs, who first elucidated the process of cells converting food into energy, which he called the citric acid cycle (CAC).

Krebs proposed a specific metabolic pathway within the cells to account for the oxidation of the basic components of food—carbohydrates, proteins, and fats—into energy. The Krebs cycle occurs inside the mitochondria—the cell's power plants—where oxygen is used to convert fuel from glucose or ketones into ATP, the energy that powers every cellular function. During this process, carbon molecules from food are broken down through a series of reactions that generate ATP, allowing the body to produce usable energy efficiently.

When excess electrons combine with oxygen, they can damage mitochondria and trigger programmed cell death. Mitochondrial uncoupling helps prevent this by allowing energy to be released without overproducing ATP. This matters because excessive ATP production increases reactive oxygen species (ROS), leading to oxidative stress that damages mitochondria and cells. In the "uncoupling to survive" hypothesis, the weakening of ROS by partial uncoupling while still maintaining sufficient ATP production can help delay cellular death.[2] How does all this tie into the Keto Flex program? Ketones are signaling molecules that not only create new mitochondria but also activate this uncoupling process.

The mitochondria are so important that the cells most needed for survival (in terms of energy-production needs) have more mitochondria. Minerals and amino acids fuel these mitochondria. Our body makes amino acids, but we need to obtain the minerals from eating the right nutrient-dense foods.

Besides producing energy for our cells, mitochondria also identify cellular threats, which can be physical, mental, emotional, or chemical.

When they perceive a threat, they produce less energy to protect the cells from harm. This is called the cell danger response, and if it continues, it can disturb our metabolism, gut microbiome, and organ systems, potentially resulting in disease and the onset of all those symptoms mentioned in the Introduction.

So, how do we keep our mitochondria functioning at optimal performance? We enter a state of ketosis. Allow me to explain. Your cells have two main energy sources: sugar (glucose) and fat (ketones). When your body breaks down carbohydrates (sugar) for energy, it doesn't produce as much energy as when it breaks down fats. Here's how it works: First, there's a process called glycolysis, which converts one molecule of glucose into two molecules of pyruvic acid (or pyruvate). Glycolysis gives you four units of energy (the ATP mentioned earlier), but it actually uses two ATPs to get going. So, in the end, you have a net gain of only two ATPs.

Next comes oxidative phosphorylation, also known as the electron transport chain (ETC). This is where the hydrogen produced during glucose metabolism gets used up. It's also where the most energy in the form of ATP is made. The ETC gives you roughly 30 ATPs. But there are still four hydrogen atoms left over, which get released and give you around two more ATPs. So, altogether, from one molecule of glucose, you get about 30 to 32 ATPs.

Now, if we look at the energy released, one ATP has about 12,000 calories (or 12 kcals). So, 32 ATPs would be around 384,000 calories, or 384 kcals. However, if you burn one gram of glucose completely, it releases about 686,000 calories, or 686 kcals. So, the efficiency of this energy transfer is about 66 percent, with the remaining 34 percent being released as heat.

Now let's switch gears and look at fat metabolism: Instead of glucose, we have palmitic acid, which is a type of saturated fat with 16 carbon atoms. First, the fatty acid needs to be activated by adding CoA to form fatty acyl-CoA. This step uses up energy (ATP). Then the fatty acyl-CoA is transported into the mitochondria with the help of carnitine. Finally, beta-oxidation takes place, where acyl-CoA goes through a series of reactions to form acetyl-CoA, which can enter the TCA cycle for more energy production. The TCA cycle (aka the Krebs cycle we discussed earlier) is your cell's energy engine. Inside the mitochondria, it takes the broken-down pieces of food—mainly acetyl-CoA from fats or carbs—and runs them through a circular series of reactions that strip away electrons. Those electrons then fuel the electron transport chain to make ATP, your body's main energy currency.

Palmitic acid and stearic acid are both natural saturated fats, but stearic acid has two more carbons, making it a bit more stable and generally healthier for your metabolism. Stearic acid, with 18 carbon atoms, provides approximately 146 ATPs. Larger fatty acids, like those with 20 carbon atoms, yield even more ATPs, around 163. Remember, one glucose molecule produces only around 30 to 32 ATPs. Palmitic acid, containing 16 carbon atoms, generates approximately 129 ATPs. So, to put it simply, burning fat for energy is like driving a sleek Porsche because it gives you more ATPs compared to burning sugar, which is more like driving an old, worn-out Toyota Corolla.[3]

During times of food shortfall or fasting—even for short periods overnight—amino acids can be converted via the Krebs cycle to glucose for energy or for storage as glycogen and fat. Our bodies can create ketones for energy whenever we need it. If we're fasting—or even during sleep—our liver produces more ketones when our insulin dips and our body shifts to fat oxidation. The three ketones produced are acetone (expelled in the breath), acetoacetate (expelled in the urine), and beta-hydroxybutyrate (BHB, expelled in the blood). Ketosis is a metabolic process that has been around for as long as humans have existed. It has literally helped our species survive. Supporting our mitochondria is the key to health and longevity, and ketosis plays an important role.

Gluconeogenesis, converting noncarbohydrate sources like lactate into glucose, supplements energy production, especially during physical exercise. A great analogy Dr. Jason Fung, best-selling author of *The Obesity Code*, shared on the *Metabolic Freedom* podcast is to think of your glycogen stores as your wallet. The cash inside your wallet represents your glucose reserves, and the benefit of using this source of energy is easy access. You can easily grab your wallet to pull out cash when you need it. The drawback is that you have a limited capacity for how much cash you can store. Your glycogen stores are similar in that they can store about 2,000 calories. Anything more will be pushed into fat cells, leading to weight gain. This might sound like a good option as the primary source of energy, but it's not. When you're relying on your sugar reserves for energy, you'd have to eat every few hours just to replenish your stores. Otherwise, your energy levels crash, and you end up feeling "hangry" (hungry and angry). Dave Asprey, best-selling author of *The Bulletproof Diet*, calls this "hypo-glybitchy." It's not fun being a sugar burner.

In contrast, think of your fat stores as your bank safe. The drawback is that it takes longer to gain access to your bank safe versus your wallet. You have to drive to the bank and wait in line. The benefit is that there are unlimited reserves in your bank safe. Similarly, you can store hundreds of thousands of calories of body fat in your body. For example, someone who has 10 percent body fat, which is very lean, has enough calories in the form of body fat to go several days without food and still survive. The goal here is to achieve the metabolic switch of burning through our glycogen stores (the wallet) so that our metabolism can start burning our fat cells (the bank safe). When carbohydrate stores are significantly decreased, the liver makes up the shortfall through increased production of ketone bodies.

HORMONES: YOUR CHEMICAL MESSENGERS

The complex chemical activities of the body are controlled by the endocrine system and the central nervous system. The endocrine system does its part by secreting hormones into the bloodstream. These secretions come from a variety of endocrine glands, which are special groups of cells. The major endocrine glands are the pituitary, pineal, thymus, thyroid, adrenal glands, and pancreas. In addition, men produce hormones in their testes and women produce them in their ovaries.

There are hundreds of hormones in your body. The key functions of hormones are to regulate the metabolic functions of the body (energy level, reproduction, growth and development, and response to injury, stress, and environmental factors); control the rate of chemical reactions in various cells; and influence the ability of substances to transport themselves through cell membranes. Because this book is focused on diet and nutrition, we'll focus on the hormones that impact those important areas.

Glucocorticoid Hormones

Your body has natural daily cycles called the circadian rhythm. Many functions—falling asleep at night, waking up, eating, and going to the bathroom—are patterned around a repeating 24-hour cycle. To prompt the body to do these things at the right time, hormones rise and fall at specific times during the day. When you interfere with these natural circadian rhythms, your health may suffer. Disrupted circadian rhythms have been linked to obesity, sleep disorders, depression, and other major health problems.

For example, a group of steroid hormones known as glucocorticoid hormones are secreted on a 12-hour cycle. These hormones drive fat-cell production from precursors.

Disrupting this cycle is linked to obesity. Some people have diseases such as Cushing's disorder, or they undergo steroid treatments that result in boosted levels of these hormones in the body and are also linked to obesity.

In addition to this natural daily rhythm, your body also secretes glucocorticoids during stressful situations. Immediately after a stressful event is experienced, there is a corticotropin-releasing hormone mediated suppression of food intake. This diverts the body's resources away from the less important need to consume food and toward prioritizing fight, flight, or withdrawal behaviors. But then, as the stressful event fades into memory, the opposite happens: There is a glucocorticoid-mediated stimulation of hunger and eating behavior.

Sex Hormones: Estrogen, Progesterone, and Testosterone

The relationship between hormone balance and weight regulation is particularly crucial in women. Even minor fluctuations in hormones can have a big impact on metabolism, which in turn can affect your weight.[4] One common issue is that as women age, certain key hormone levels decrease, making weight gain more likely. Later in the book, you'll discover how to follow a ketogenic and fasting approach customized to women who are at different stages of life (cycling and perimenopausal or postmenopausal).

Women who are experiencing perimenopause and menopause will see their estrogen levels drop.[5] The body then looks for estrogen held in fat cells, which spurs the body to make more fat to make up for the estrogen shortfall.

Progesterone is an endogenous steroid involved in the menstrual cycle, pregnancy, and embryogenesis. It's produced mainly in the ovaries following ovulation each month. As women age, progesterone levels also decrease. With a progesterone deficit comes that puffy, bloated feeling that accompanies water retention.

Most people think of testosterone as a male sex hormone, but everyone requires a certain amount. Testosterone helps build muscle and burn calories. While males have more testosterone than females, female adrenal glands and ovaries produce small amounts. Women lose testosterone during menopause, which leads to muscle loss, lower metabolism, and weight gain.

Cortisol, Stress, and Belly Fat

Cortisol is one of the steroid hormones and is made in the adrenal glands. It helps regulate metabolism, control blood sugar levels, reduce inflammation, assist with memory formulation, and control blood pressure, and it has a stabilizing effect on salt and water balance. Elevated levels of cortisol due to stress have been linked to weight gain, and particularly the accumulation of abdominal fat. Stress-induced abdominal fat is unhealthy because it secretes large amounts of inflammatory molecules that contribute to insulin resistance, diabetes, and heart attacks.

Your body can't distinguish between the stress produced by a lion chasing you and being stuck in a traffic jam. This is why it's imperative to master stress so that it's not chronically elevated, leading to a host of symptoms. Stress is the silent killer that we all need to be aware of.

Hunger and Satiety Hormones: Ghrelin and Leptin

Our bodies have appetite- and weight-regulating hormones that strive to maintain homeostasis (that is, a steady hormonal "set point") throughout the day. When we take in less food energy than we expend through basal metabolism and activity, our bodies respond by trying to correct the problem and make us hungry. Two vital hormones that modulate our appetite and hunger signals are ghrelin and leptin.

Ghrelin is a hormone that increases appetite and plays a role in body weight. I compare ghrelin to a gremlin because it makes noise and it's not fun when it's around. Ghrelin encourages you to pick up the fork. It's released primarily in the lining of the stomach, goes into the blood, crosses the blood-brain barrier, and arrives at your hypothalamus, where it tells you you're hungry. Researchers have suggested that ghrelin levels influence how quickly hunger returns after you eat.

Leptin is a hormone secreted primarily in fat cells, as well as the stomach, heart, placenta, and skeletal muscle. It travels to the hypothalamus and signals that you have enough fat, so you can eat less or stop eating. It decreases your appetite so you put down the fork. Leptin may also increase metabolism, although there is unresolved research on this point.

Leptin production correlates to fat mass—the more fat you have, the more leptin you produce. Your leptin levels are lower if you're thin and higher if you're heavyset. You would think that having more leptin would help you lose weight because it suppresses your appetite. The problem is that many obese people have built up a resistance to the appetite-suppressing effects of leptin. Once you arrive at a certain "fat mass," your excess body fat will disrupt your appetite signals and make you hungrier. Essentially, obesity can disrupt normal appetite signaling so that signals from leptin and ghrelin may not always work in the expected ways.

Overall, research suggests that ghrelin production seems to be affected by growth hormone release, which differs in men and women. Dr. Sylvia Tara's book, *The Secret Life of Fat*, shows research on women producing 33 percent more ghrelin than men after exercise. Leptin seems to influence fertility and reproduction in women, which are related to women's body-fat levels. Women appear to be more sensitive than men to leptin levels. This is a perfect example of why women practice health differently than men, and why an entire chapter in this book is customized for you ladies.

Sleep is another factor. A lack of sleep results in less leptin and more ghrelin—which increases your appetite—as well as disrupted glucose and insulin metabolism.[6] Cortisol levels are also higher when you don't get adequate sleep, which may then increase appetite. This can become a vicious cycle, which is why you must prioritize healthy sleep to maximize the Keto Flex lifestyle.

Research has repeatedly shown that inadequate sleep is linked to weight gain and a higher body mass index (BMI). While people's sleep requirements vary, short sleep duration increases the likelihood of obesity in both children and adults. Weight gain has been seen in experimental sleep-deprivation studies, and the reward centers of the brain are more stimulated by food when you're sleep deprived. Poor sleep can increase the brain's pleasurable response to food and decrease your self-control and decision-making abilities. To make the problem even worse, many sleep disorders, such as sleep apnea, are exacerbated by weight gain. It's a vicious cycle that can be difficult to break: Poor sleep can cause weight gain, which can then worsen sleep quality, triggering more weight gain.

The Environmental Impact on Your Hormones

Scientists are still researching the way the environment impacts our hormones, from substances in plastics (like BPA) to flame retardants in fabrics, furniture, curtains, and carpets. Chemicals in the environment known as endocrine disruptors may affect our body's endocrine system by mimicking naturally occurring hormones. In response, our body may respond by overproducing or underproducing the mimicked hormones and others. Endocrine disruptors have been linked with developmental, reproductive, brain, immune, and other problems. Even low doses of endocrine-disrupting chemicals may be unsafe. The body's normal endocrine functioning involves slight changes in hormone levels, and we know even these small changes can cause significant developmental and biological effects. Studies have shown a link between these toxins and obesity, leading scientists to label them "obesogens."

Environmental toxins are making us sick and fat.

Some toxins are worse than others. I believe the four biggest toxins creating inflammation in our world are the heavy metals lead and mercury, mold toxicity, and glyphosate.

So, what can we do to protect ourselves from all these toxins in our environment? The first step is to do an audit in your home. Replace any household items that you suspect are problematic with nontoxic, natural alternatives. My favorite nontoxic brands—the ones I personally use and trust—include dōTERRA, Truly Free (for nontoxic detergents), Dr. Bronner's, MamaSuds, Branch Basics, and Natural Choice Company. Each of these companies is dedicated to creating clean, safe, and effective products that support a toxin-free home and a healthier body.

Supporting your liver is also key for eliminating environmental toxins. Cytochrome P450 is composed of 50 different enzymes, and while they are found in all tissues of the body, the highest concentration is within liver cells, which are essential during phase 1 of liver detoxification. As the primary site of drug metabolism, the liver functions to detoxify and facilitate excretion of xenobiotics (foreign drugs or chemicals) by enzymatically converting lipid-soluble compounds to more water-soluble compounds. This process is micronutrient dependent. Daily toxins deplete your micronutrients. If you are micronutrient deficient, then it's likely your detoxification pathways aren't working properly.

If your detoxification pathways are constantly being used to do the job of dealing with these toxins, they aren't available to perform other fat-burning jobs, such as creating brown adipose tissue, which is crucial for maintaining core body temperature and energy balance. Keep your minerals up and support your liver. You'll learn later in the book why we love bitters for the liver, and how keto and fasting help to reverse conditions such as fatty liver disease.

▲▼▲

Wow, that was a lot of science! Hopefully now you understand why healthy cells are a foundation for overall health and why it's so important to fuel them with the right sources of energy. These energy sources also affect the function of our hormones, which play a critical role in regulating our weight, metabolism, and more to keep us in optimal health. You know what else has an incredible impact on our health? Fasting. And in the next chapter, we'll look at some of the surprising benefits.

CHAPTER TWO

HOW FASTING SAVES THE DAY (AND YOUR WAISTLINE)

Even though fasting has been clinically proven to be effective, fasting naysayers still exist. The most common criticism is that it's too "stressful" for your body. While fasting is a stress to your body, that's not necessarily a bad thing. Saying you shouldn't fast because it's too stressful to your body is like saying you shouldn't exercise because it's too stressful for your body. Stress is bad only if your body does not adapt properly. Stress is vital for health and longevity when your body adapts to the stressors. Sometimes fasting is the key to keto success. Let's take my client John, for example.

For years John felt trapped in an endless cycle. While he was athletic growing up, over the years his weight had spiraled upward—at his heaviest he weighed 446 pounds. He could no longer wear jeans, because they didn't make them in his size, and climbing stairs at his UPS job left him in agony. He'd been working to lose weight, but he hit a wall when he reached 308 pounds. He was following a keto diet, yet for months he remained stuck at that weight. Eventually the frustration would overwhelm him, and he'd crash—cheating for three or four days, gaining back 10 to 12 pounds, and then returning to strict dieting for another few months. When John found my Keto Flex program, he was 58 years old, and he made a commitment to follow my protocol exactly—no cheating. By the end of 30 days, John had lost 44 pounds. But his transformation went beyond weight loss: His knee pain vanished, the inflammation throughout his body disappeared, and he felt confident again. Following the ketogenic diet, drinking the Keto Kamp Cocktail, walking after meals, and doing the intermittent-fasting protocols all worked together to finally break his frustrating plateau.

In this chapter I'll explain how this type of "good" stress works, and the difference between fasting and starving. We'll look at ancient fasting and how physicians have used this as a tool for thousands of years to help cure illness. Even today, therapeutic fasting has been implemented to improve certain health conditions.

HORMESIS—AKA GOOD STRESS

Hormesis is one of the most important principles I have learned about health. It's when a small amount of a harmful substance provides beneficial effects for our body. Exercise is the easiest example of how hormesis works. If you've been inactive for 10 years and you decide to do a high-intensity workout at the gym, your body will have a hard time adapting to that much stress. But if instead you slowly build up your workout, starting out with a walk on the treadmill and some light weights, your body will adapt to this stress and grow stronger. Over time you can gradually increase this stress, stay in your "hormetic zone," and experience the added benefits.

Fasting also stresses your body, but it's a bad stress only when you don't properly adapt to the stress. When you stay in your hormetic zone, you achieve incredible results.

How do you know if you're adapting to the stress of fasting? Track your blood glucose and ketones during your fast using a Keto-Mojo device. (You can purchase this over at benazadi.com/ketomojo.) You want to see your blood glucose gradually dropping while your blood ketones are gradually increasing. If you see the opposite trend, it's time to break the fast and try again sometime soon. Another great metric to see if fasting is working for you or against you is heart rate variability (HRV). HRV is highly individual—genetics influence your baseline, so the key is to identify your personal average and focus on gradually improving it over time. HRV is probably the best marker to assess the health of your nervous system. You have two primary branches of your nervous system: the parasympathetic branch, which is your rest, digest, relax, and detoxification system; and your sympathetic branch, which is your flight-or-fight response that produces adrenaline and cortisol. The goal is to have a healthy balance of both. Find your baseline and work on increasing HRV. If you see your HRV drop below your average and it was a longer-than-usual fasting day, this could signal that your fast was too stressful on the body. I personally use the Oura ring to track my HRV. Other devices, such as the WHOOP band and Ultrahuman ring, also track HRV.

During your 45-Day Keto Flex Reset, each step is designed to get you ready for fasting techniques so your body adapts and stays within the hormetic zone.

FASTING VS. STARVING

The first, and most important, distinction to make is between fasting and starving. Starving is what happens when, *against your will,* your access to food is restricted or shut off, causing your health to suffer, and perhaps even leading to death. Sadly, throughout human history, starvation has been a constant problem, even today. Fasting is when, in an environment where food is readily available, you *choose* to restrict your food intake in order to achieve a rational goal.

The Guinness World Record for the longest recorded fast went to Angus Barbieri, a Scotsman who went 382 days without food. His starting weight was 472 pounds, and his ending weight was 178pounds. He was medically supervised, and doctors tracked his electrolytes and blood work throughout. It's been reported that Angus had coffee, tea, and a multivitamin, but no actual meal during the entire 382 days. I would argue that while Angus didn't put food in his mouth for 382 days, he was "eating" from his body fat. He had a lot of fuel to consume!

FASTING WITH A HISTORY OF AN EATING DISORDER

Eating disorders are when someone has an unhealthy relationship to food and eating has become intertwined with a deeply rooted psychological problem. It may be difficult for others to understand this, but to the person with an eating disorder, their extreme actions represent an *agreeable solution* to a more painful psychological problem and bring very real emotional relief. The following are some common eating disorders:

- **Anorexia nervosa** is characterized by a distorted body image springing from an unfounded fear of being overweight. Patients literally see themselves as fat even when self-starvation has made them emaciated.
- **Binge-eating disorder** typically takes the form of eating unusually large amounts of food in relatively short periods of time and feeling a lack of control during binges.
- **Bulimia nervosa** involves secret bingeing—eating large amounts of food with a loss of control over the eating—followed by purging in an effort to get rid of the unwanted calories in an unhealthy way. Methods of purging include forced vomiting, excessive use of laxatives or diuretics, and extreme or prolonged periods of exercising.
- **Pica** is an eating disorder that involves eating things that are not considered food. People with pica crave and ingest nonfood substances such as ice, soap, pebbles, paper, dirt, hair, cloth, soil, chalk, laundry detergent, wool, or cornstarch.
- **Rumination disorder** is a condition in which a person regurgitates food they have previously chewed and swallowed, rechews it, and then either re-swallows it or spits it out. Rumination disorder can result in weight loss and severe malnutrition that can be fatal.
- **Orthorexia**—not yet recognized as a separate eating disorder by the current *Diagnostic and Statistical Manual of Mental Disorders* (DSM)—manifests itself as an obsessive focus on healthy eating with no rational

reason or goal. The affected person may eliminate entire food groups, leading to malnutrition, difficulty eating outside the home, severe weight loss, and emotional distress. Their self-worth, identity, or satisfaction is dependent upon how well they comply with their irrational, self-imposed diet rules.

All these disorders require mental health counseling or psychiatric treatment and can take years to resolve. Note that none of them involve setting a rational goal and then working to meet that goal; they are all about a morbid relationship with food, stemming from a deep-seated emotional problem. I do not recommend fasting for anyone currently struggling with an eating disorder.

ANCIENT FASTING

Fasting has a long and storied history. The Bible makes frequent references to fasting. In the Old Testament, fasting fell into two categories: private and public. Private fasts were seen as acts of personal penance, while prayer, supplication, and sackcloth accompanied public fasts. When Moses ascended Mount Sinai to receive the Ten Commandments, he fasted as an act of self-purification: "So he was there with the Lord forty days and forty nights. He neither ate bread nor drank water. And he wrote on the tablets the words of the covenant, the Ten Commandments" (Exodus 34:28, English Standard Version).

And when John the Baptist lived in the desert, he subsisted on a very restricted diet: "Now John wore a garment of camel's hair and a leather belt around his waist, and his food was locusts and wild honey" (Matthew 3:4, ESV). But wait—he lived on locusts and wild honey? When you think about it, that's a nutritionally complete diet. Locusts are about 50 percent protein, 19 percent fat, 16 percent crude fiber, 5 percent carbs, and 10 percent water. They're a good source of iodine, phosphorus, iron, thiamine, riboflavin, and niacin, and have traces of calcium, magnesium, and selenium. Honey is mainly fructose (about 38 percent) and glucose (about 32 percent), with remaining sugars including maltose, sucrose, and other complex carbohydrates.

If John the Baptist ate mostly locusts, with a bit of honey now and then as a treat, and if he had access to a daily multivitamin pill, he would have been very close to a healthy ketogenic diet!

Since self-imposed fasting involves exercising control of the physical body, many religions consider fasting a way to cultivate mental discipline and use it in connection with prayer or meditation to heighten the spiritual experience and demonstrate adherence to custom. Fasting is particularly important for Christians during Lent and Muslims during the holy month of Ramadan. Yogic practices, including that of fasting, date back thousands of years. In the 20th century, Paramahansa Yogananda said, "Fasting is a natural method of healing."[1] In the Bahá'í faith, strict fasting—the complete abstention from both food and drink—is observed from sunrise to sunset during the Bahá'í month of 'Alá', from March 2 through March 20. In Judaism, while Yom Kippur is the only fast day that is explicitly stated in the Torah, observant Jews fast six days of the year. On Yom Kippur, fasting as a means of repentance is mandatory for every Jewish man and boy above the bar mitzvah age and every Jewish woman and girl above the bat mitzvah age.

In the Greek and Roman eras, we see fasting used not only as a method of spiritual cleansing but also as a way to combat disease. It's important to remember that ancient "physicians" (if you can call them that) had no way of knowing the inner workings of a living human being. They had knowledge of anatomy from cadavers, but many basic organ functions, particularly those of the heart and the brain, were unknown. The causes of infectious disease—viruses and bacteria—were unknown. All they had was careful observation of human behavior under various conditions.

In the 5th century BCE, Greek physician Hippocrates recommended abstinence from food or drink for patients who exhibited symptoms of certain illnesses. He and other natural philosophers recognized that patients in certain disease states naturally experienced a loss of appetite. Since fasting was thought to be an important natural part of the recovery process, administering food during such states was unnecessary and possibly even harmful because you were fueling the disease. Hippocrates wrote, "To eat when you are sick is to feed your illness."

Around the same time, it was written that when the Buddha was traveling in the region of Kasi, near present-day Varanasi, India, he addressed a sangha of monks, saying, "I, monks, do not eat a meal in the evening. Not eating a meal in the evening, I, monks, am aware of good health and of being without illness and of buoyancy and strength and living in comfort. Come, do you too, monks, not eat a meal in the evening. Not eating a meal in the evening, you too, monks, will be aware of good health and . . . living in comfort."[2] And that's how the tradition of Buddhist monks avoiding food intake after noon was born.

Five centuries after Buddha and Hippocrates, Plutarch wrote, "Instead of using medicine, better fast today."[3] Fifteen hundred years later, Philip Paracelsus, the Swiss founder of the science of toxicology during the German Renaissance, wrote, "Fasting is the greatest remedy—the physician within."[4] And good ol' Benjamin Franklin, one of America's Founding Fathers and a man who knew a lot about a wide variety of topics, said, "The best of all medicines is resting and fasting."[5] Even today, we all know the common axiom "Feed a cold, starve a fever."

THERAPEUTIC FASTING

In the United States, therapeutic fasting, intended to treat illness or maintain good health, became popular in the 19th century as part of the natural hygiene movement. Much of the health and nutrition advice many people follow today—the role of fasting in the recovery of health, the advantages of a plant-based diet, the incredible healing powers of the body, and the importance of avoiding unnecessary drugs and surgery—were promoted by natural hygienists as far back as 150 years ago.

In 1928, Dr. Herbert Shelton (1895–1985) opened Dr. Shelton's Health School in San Antonio, Texas. He claimed to have helped 40,000 patients recover their health with a water fast. Nominated in 1956 by the American Vegetarian Party as candidate for President of the United States, he wrote, "Fasting must be recognized as a fundamental and radical process that is older than any other mode of caring for the sick organism, for it is employed on the plane of instinct."[6]

In natural medicine, fasting is seen as a way of cleansing the body of toxins, removing diseased or dead tissues, and giving the digestive system a chance to reset to homeostasis. Such fasts typically allow only water, or sometimes clear fruit and vegetable juices. Fasting has also been used in the treatment of some kinds of cancer, autoimmune diseases, and allergies. There are a ton of research studies showing how effective fasting can be for you.

In their 2019 study entitled "Ten-Hour Time-Restricted Eating Reduces Weight, Blood Pressure, and Atherogenic Lipids in Patients with Metabolic Syndrome," Dr. Pam Taub, a cardiologist at the University of California, San Diego School of Medicine and her colleagues tested a group of subjects who had metabolic syndrome. This means they all showed a cluster of conditions that occur together, including increased blood pressure, high blood sugar, excess body fat around the waist, and abnormal cholesterol or triglyceride levels. Metabolic disorder increases the risk of heart disease, stroke, and type 2 diabetes. The 19 participants underwent 10 hours of time-restricted eating (TRE)—all dietary intake within a consistent self-selected 10-hour window—for 12 weeks. The researchers found this TRE intervention improved participants' cardiometabolic health and concluded, "TRE is a potentially powerful lifestyle intervention that can be added to standard medical practice to treat metabolic syndrome."[7]

In the study, participants experienced an average 3 percent reduction in body weight and a 4 percent reduction in abdominal visceral fat. The researchers also reported improvements in cholesterol levels, blood pressure, and sleep quality, with many participants noting increased energy.

The authors explained that fasting depletes the body's glucose stores and shifts metabolism toward fat utilization, allowing the body to enter a low-grade state of ketosis.[1]

Remember, these participants did a TRE of 10 hours, with 14 hours of fasting, and they didn't eat a special diet. Imagine the results they—and you—could get with the Keto Flex lifestyle over a longer period of time!

Even if you don't need to lose weight, intermittent fasting is a health booster! In a 2018 study entitled "Early Time-Restricted Feeding Improves Insulin Sensitivity, Blood Pressure, and Oxidative Stress Even

Without Weight Loss in Men with Prediabetes," researchers conducted a supervised, controlled feeding trial to determine whether intermittent fasting (IF) had benefits independent of weight loss by feeding participants enough food to maintain their weight. They used early time-restricted feeding (eTRF), a form of IF that involves eating early in the day to be in alignment with circadian rhythms in metabolism. They found that male subjects with prediabetes showed improvements in insulin sensitivity, β-cell responsiveness, blood pressure, oxidative stress, and appetite. They demonstrated that eTRF improved cardiometabolic health and that IF's effects were not solely due to weight loss.[8]

Research has shown that fasting can help with:

- reducing high blood pressure;[9]
- digestive health (including acid reflux, gas, bloating, puffiness, GERD, diarrhea, leaky gut, and autoimmune conditions);
- intestinal stem cell regeneration;[10]
- microbe diversity in the gut;[11]
- cancer prevention;[12] and
- increasing metabolism.[13]

If you're interested in learning more of the details about how fasting can improve all the above, see my book *Metabolic Freedom*.

FASTING FOR BRAIN HEALTH

Our brain *function* doesn't decrease when we fast, but our brain *energy* does. According to research by Thomas DeLauer, author, health expert, and performance coach, the "slowing down" of synaptic activity is the brain's way of conserving energy and giving itself a chance to recharge. This means the brain becomes more efficient. If you normally have 100 percent energy in your brain when you're eating a normal diet and not fasting, it will be diversified throughout multiple areas of your brain. In terms of synaptic energy, let's say you need to process 10 things. You have 100 percent brainpower, and you're allocating 10 percent to each of 10 different areas of your brain. But when you're fasting, your body becomes more efficient and turns off mechanisms that don't need to be used. So, even if your overall brain energy is now 50 percent instead of 100 percent, that 50 percent is focused on one area at a time. This is why you can feel so much more alert with the task at hand when you're fasting. We were hardwired this way when we were hunter-gatherers, because we had to be focused and sharp to catch our next meal. I would rather have 50 percent less energy and have that energy focused on where I want it than have 100 percent energy scattered all over the place in areas I don't really need.

When we're fasting, we're also not producing nearly as many neurotransmitters like serotonin and dopamine, among others. While these neurotransmitters are important, they are metabolically costly to produce, meaning they're not exactly the best use of our body's energy. We often produce more than we need. If we reduced the number of neurotransmitters being produced like we did with the synaptic activity, it would take a load off the central nervous system and allow us to be more efficient and productive with how we use those neurotransmitters.

By reducing the release of neurotransmitters from synapses in the brain, fasting may also give the nervous system a break. It's also worth noting that high levels of synaptic activity (overactive synaptic activity) and high levels of neurotransmitter production are associated with neurodegenerative diseases, including Alzheimer's, Huntington's, and Parkinson's.

When we're fasting, we also produce more brain-derived neurotrophic factor, or BDNF, which grows neurons and strengthens synaptic connectivity, making it easier for neurons to communicate. Put it this way: If you have two neurons that are communicating with each other, and you have a high amount of activity but a low-quality connection, you're basically trying to cram 10 percent of that energy across a broken bridge where things are sliding off and the activity is falling through the cracks. When you're fasting, however, you have more neural connectivity with more efficient synaptic activity. Now with 50 percent of your energy going across a good, sturdy, unbroken, and structured bridge, the communication will surely get from neuron to neuron. BDNF also interacts with neurons in the hippocampus, cortex, and basal forebrain, all areas involved in memory, focus, and overall sense of well-being.

▲▼▲

Fasting has been used for thousands of years to encourage healing in the body, and now, in modern times, we have the research to prove its effectiveness in the treatment of various health conditions. As we'll see in the pages ahead, when used as part of the Keto Flex lifestyle, intermittent, deliberate fasting can be an easy way (what's easier than *not* eating?) to clean out our reserves of glucose, burn ketones, lose weight, and feel great.

CHAPTER THREE

KETOSIS: WHEN BUTTER IS THE BEST PRESCRIPTION

The word *diet* strikes fear into the hearts of most people. Let's be honest, do *you* like the word *diet*? When we hear that word, most of us conjure up images of deprivation and frustration. We immediately think of all the foods we won't be allowed to eat as well as the potential hunger pangs from consuming less food. We wonder if it will be worth the time and struggle—or if we'll ultimately just regain whatever weight we lose. To most people who have tried to lose weight by dieting, the whole idea seems like an exercise in misery and failure—and statistics support this impression. That's why my goal with this chapter is to make the case for keto as a *metabolic process*, not a diet.

In this chapter I'll explain why the way our brains are wired makes it difficult for traditional diets to work. Our primal brains are so programmed for survival that they begin to panic when we lose body fat. I'll also share the many extraordinary benefits of a ketogenic lifestyle, from improving polycystic ovary syndrome (PCOS) symptoms to targeting cancer cells. A Keto Flex lifestyle can even help us live longer!

DIETS DON'T LAST

A 2020 study in the *BMJ*, the weekly peer-reviewed medical trade journal published by the British Medical Association, examined the results of 121 random trials with nearly 22,000 patients enrolled in 14 diet plans. Each person followed a popular diet and reported weight loss and changes in cardiovascular risk factors. The diets were macronutrient or "macro," which go beyond calorie counting and track the macronutrients—grams of proteins, carbs, and fats—you're eating within your calorie goal and ratios. According to the study, evidence showed that over a period of six months, most macronutrient diets produced moderate weight loss and improvements in cardiovascular risk factors like blood pressure. Okay—so far, so good. The bad news is that after 12 months, the positive effect on weight reduction and improvements in cardiovascular risk factors largely vanished. The study's authors also made the interesting observation that "differences between diets are, however, generally trivial to small, implying that people can choose the diet they prefer from among many of the available diets without concern about the magnitude of benefits."[1]

A similar study published in *Medical Clinics of North America* in 2018 followed 29 long-term weight-loss studies, revealing that more than half of the weight lost by participants was regained within two years, and by five years, more than 80 percent of lost weight was regained. Authors Kevin Hall, PhD, and Scott Kahan, MD, noted, "Previous failed attempts at achieving durable weight loss may have contributed to the recent decrease in the percentage of people with obesity who are trying to lose weight and many now believe that weight loss is a futile endeavor."[2]

Typically, when we first start a diet, we have the most enthusiasm and willpower. But this is short-lived, and soon the diet begins to feel tedious, punitive, and impossibly hard. And there's a reason for that: Our primal brains instinctively want to maintain our weight, so over time it becomes harder and harder to resist eating the foods we crave, particularly fats.

THE TRIUNE BRAIN

When discussing the failure of diets, it's important to understand the decision-making structure of the brain. In the 1960s, American neuroscientist Paul MacLean formulated the triune brain model, which proposed that the human brain had evolved into three distinct regions, forming a hierarchy. The three regions are as follows:

1. **Reptilian or primal brain.** This is the basal ganglia, a group of structures found deep within the cerebral hemispheres. It's responsible for the fight-or-flight survival response and other primal activities related to our survival.
2. **Paleomammalian or emotional brain.** This is the limbic system, a set of middle-layer structures in the brain that deal with emotions and memory. It regulates autonomic or endocrine function in response to emotional stimuli and is involved in reinforcing behavior.
3. **Neomammalian or rational brain.** This is the neocortex, a set of outer layers involved in higher-order brain functions, including sensory perception, cognition, generation of motor commands, spatial reasoning, and language. This is the distinctly "human" part of the brain. Many other animals have robust primal and emotional brain functions.[3]

While modern brain-imaging technology has shown that MacLean's model is an oversimplification, it's useful for explaining how we humans can consciously think we should do something, and yet some inner control center in our own brain issues contradictory commands. For example, Jane wanted to lose 20 pounds. She was 40 years old and had been eating the same way her entire adult life. Little by little, the pounds crept up, and one day she decided enough was enough. She enrolled in a diet plan. Nutrisystem, Weight Watchers, Jenny Craig, Atkins—it doesn't matter which one she chose. This was a decision made by her rational brain. It said to her, "You have a weight problem, and the solution is to go on a diet. All you have to do is eat the food you're supposed to and not eat anything else, and the pounds will melt away." No problem, right? It's like choosing to drive your car at 55 mph instead of 65 mph because you know it will increase your gas mileage. Not a big deal, and you'll still get to where you're going.

Jane went on her diet. It was unpleasant because she never really felt like she had enough to eat at mealtimes. She felt deprived, her stomach growled at her, and she looked longingly at delicious food choices she couldn't have. But after a few weeks, she lost a few pounds. Her emotional brain was happy. She liked that her clothes fit better and she looked more slender. So far, so good. But deep in her reptilian primal brain, alarm bells were ringing. Something terrible was happening! Jane's calories had been cut, and the actual mass of her body was shrinking! For millions of years, the reptilian brain has been responsible for the most basic tasks of the survival of the species, and now it sensed a major threat. Whatever was happening out there in the "rational" world, it wasn't good. The weight loss conjured up primitive memories deep in her DNA of lean times and even starvation. That was unacceptable. It was time to put the brakes on this madness and *get some food*. And so, by degrees, Jane started to cheat on her diet as her reptilian brain cajoled her into eating more and restoring her body to the comfortable state it was in before she had begun her weight-loss program.

Sometimes, it's the emotional brain that pulls the plug on a diet. People eat for many reasons, not just to fill their bellies when they're hungry. Eating is bound up with all sorts of emotional baggage, and many people eat to relieve anxiety or depression. Emotional eating can suppress or soothe boredom, stress, sadness, anger, fear, and loneliness. Your emotions can become so intertwined with your eating habits that without thinking about what you're doing, whenever you're angry or stressed, you automatically reach for a delicious treat. Eating sugary foods releases dopamine in your brain. The happy effect you feel when you eat a candy bar is real. When the reward system is activated, it reinforces the behavior that triggered it, making it more likely you'll carry out these actions again. Breaking these habits can be like kicking a drug habit.

IT'S NOT YOUR FAULT

If you accept the premise that the primal brain overrides the rational brain's choice to go on a diet with restricted foods and calories, then it's easy to see how difficult it is to stay on a diet while the primal brain is fighting you every step of the way. You may *think* you want to lose weight, and you may even know you *must* lose weight for your health, but it's like rolling a giant boulder uphill: The minute you relax, the boulder hurtles right back down to the base of the hill, where it wants to be. Then you feel guilty and ashamed, and vow never to do it again . . . until a few months later, when some new diet program is advertised on television. Clearly, there are several problems with traditional weight-loss diets.

The Food Is Unsatisfying

Following the beliefs established in the 1960s, many commercial weight-loss plans adhere to a low-fat diet. They provide food that *looks* like the delicious treats you crave—even things like brownies and ice-cream sundaes—but these pathetic low-fat imitations leave you feeling cheated. Foods labeled "fat-free," "reduced fat," "low-fat," or "sugar-free" don't equate with calorie-free, and they often contain additives like chemical fillers that make them decidedly unhealthy. Reduced-fat foods also have a perceived healthy image, and studies have shown that people tend to eat much more of these foods, either because they mistakenly believe it's okay to splurge on "low-fat" foods or because the foods are so unsatisfying that they need to eat more. When you see the terms "fat-free," "sugar-free," "low-fat," "skim milk," and "all natural," think of the phrase "chemical shitstorm."

The Food Can Be Bad for Your Health

Many diet foods contain artificial sweeteners, which are universally worse for you than real sugar. When it comes to weight management, the microbiome is a huge key. Your microbiome consists of all the microbes—bacteria, fungi, protozoa, and viruses—that live on and inside your body. The microbiome may weigh as much as five pounds, with most of it in your digestive tract. You might think zero-calorie artificial sweeteners would be beneficial for weight loss, but actually they are obesogenic, meaning they contribute to obesity. They do so by altering the microbiota composition of the gut. Under the influence of artificial sweeteners, gut bacteria changes to bacteria that is much more likely to cause fat storage and obesity.

Aspartame is the world's most widely used artificial sweetener. Marketed as NutraSweet, Equal, Sugar Twin, and AminoSweet, aspartame is present in more than 6,000 products, including Diet Coke and Diet Pepsi. It is a synthetic chemical composed of the amino acids phenylalanine and aspartic acid, with a methyl ester. When it's consumed, your body breaks down the methyl ester into methanol, which may be converted into formaldehyde.

That's right—embalming fluid.

As US Right to Know pointed out, the US Food and Drug Administration first approved aspartame for some uses in 1981, saying it was "safe for the general population under certain conditions." But "many scientists, then and now, have said the approval was based on suspect data and should be reconsidered." Dozens of studies have linked aspartame to significant health risks, including mood disorders, Alzheimer's disease, headaches and migraines, cancer, seizures, intestinal dysbiosis, cardiovascular disease, stroke, and dementia.[4] Evidence also links aspartame to increased appetite, weight gain, and obesity-related diseases.[5] In fact, such evidence raises questions about the legality of marketing aspartame-containing products as "diet" drinks or weight-loss products. In April 2015, US Right to Know petitioned the Federal Trade Commission (FTC) and the Food and Drug Administration (FDA) to investigate the marketing and advertising practices of "diet" products that contain aspartame.[6]

"Grazing" Interferes with Fat Burning and Digestion

Some popular diets advise you to eat five or six small meals throughout the day. The idea behind "grazing" is that it keeps you from getting too hungry and then overeating. One of the many problems with grazing is that as you eat one snack after another, your body is constantly producing insulin. Insulin is your fat-storage hormone, which signals your body to transport the extra glucose in your blood into your fat tissues to prevent you from losing weight. Insulin is the neighborhood bully: When he comes around, all of your fat-burning hormones scatter. And each time you eat, you have an opportunity to overeat, even by a little bit. It's one more opportunity to make a bad choice.

Another problem is that your gut is designed to "reset" after a meal, and a series of muscular contractions "sweeps" your small intestine from your stomach. This series of motions or contractions is called *peristalsis*. Each time you eat, the sweeping motion starts again from the top. If you keep introducing food into the system, your small intestine never experiences a full wave of cleaning.

Although the large intestine also has peristalsis like the small intestine, general contractions called "mass movements" occur one to three times per day, propelling what is now feces toward the rectum. Mass movements are triggered by meals, as the presence of food being digested in the stomach and duodenum (the first part of the small intestine) prompts them. This is called the gastrocolic reflex, which controls the motility of the lower gastrointestinal tract following a meal in response to the stretch of the stomach with the ingestion of food. If you eat many small meals, your stomach never stretches, which will disrupt your gastrocolic reflex.

Dental Health

While it's not a direct concern of this book, if you graze all day, you'll need to be committed to brushing your teeth after every snack. Really? Can you do that? I'll bet not. Having a coating of food on your teeth and gums all day is a ticket to cavities, gum disease, and bad breath. I've also seen upstream issues with the mouth factor into health results, including cavitations (holes in the jawbone) from tooth extractions, infected root canals, and mercury fillings. I highly recommend you listen to episodes one and two of the *Metabolic Freedom* podcast to learn more. Seek out a biological dentist in your area to explore these issues. A great resource is IAOMT.org.

BURNING SUGAR VS. BURNING FAT

As discussed earlier, the body can burn only two types of fuel: fat and sugar. Regardless of the specific foods you choose to eat, the goal is to regularly enter into a state of ketosis, where your body is burning fat for fuel instead of sugar.

Most people who consume the standard American diet (SAD) are pure sugar burners. Their food intake produces a steady enlargement of fat cells, and this fat is never used for fuel. A sugar burner is someone who relies on glucose as the main source of fuel. When you're burning sugar, your brain is going to signal intense cravings for carbohydrate-rich foods. It's really not your fault—it's your default setting right now.

You may point out that if you consumed nothing but the fat in your body as fuel, the end result would be starvation and death. This is exactly what happens to people during periods of extreme famine. Following total food deprivation, the effects of starvation (which we do not want) come in two stages:

1. **Consumption of stored sugar.** Your body can store about 2,000 calories of sugar in the form of glycogen. Skeletal muscles store about 400 grams of glycogen, and the liver stores 90 to 110 grams of glycogen. As you can imagine, in an active person, 2,000 calories lasts less than a day. Then it's depleted.
2. **Ketosis.** The body uses stored fat for energy. The breakdown occurs in the liver and turns fat into ketones. This phase, which is good, can last for weeks at a time. After fasting has gone on for one week, your brain will use these ketones and any leftover glucose. Using ketones lowers your need for glucose, and your body slows down the breakdown of proteins. Eventually starvation occurs, because you are not consuming more food.

As you'll see in the pages ahead, the goal is to become metabolically flexible (hence "flex") by going back and forth between sugar burning and fat burning. You build up a little bit of fat, and then you burn it for fuel—just like putting food in your freezer and taking it out a week later. You don't just leave it there forever!

WHY THE KETO FLEX METHOD IS GOOD FOR YOUR HEALTH

If you look at all the evidence, including how we have eaten over thousands of years and how our digestive system is designed, you have to conclude that for optimum efficiency and good health, intermittent fasting combined with a diet high in natural fats and protein (and low in carbohydrates) is the way to go. The body is accustomed to using ketones as fuel, and it's been doing that for millions of years.

Of course, many people have questions about intermittent fasting, mostly fueled by all the myths about it—that if you fast, your body will cannibalize your muscles, or that your brain will shut down, or you'll feel so starved that the minute your fast ends, you'll gorge on too much food. These stories are all nonsense, and if you try intermittent fasting, you'll quickly find out for yourself. The previous chapter on the science of fasting hopefully convinced you to use it as a health tool.

But what about the myths floating around about keto? As you'll see, keto actually has a positive effect on many symptoms and diseases, including PCOS, obesity, epilepsy, Alzheimer's, Parkinson's, cancer, acne, diabetes, autism, cardiovascular disease, high blood pressure, and fatty liver disease.

Ketosis Stresses Your Body

You might think the above statement is a negative one, but as we learned about with the process of hormesis earlier, not all stress is bad. Ketosis has been shown to trigger autophagy, which is the recycling of damaged cells and cell components. This paired with fasting is a significant way to harness your innate intelligence for fat loss, because autophagy will get rid of the bad cells that struggle to use fat as energy so you can fat-adapt faster and make ketones sooner.

Keto for Brain Disorders: Alzheimer's, Dementia, Parkinson's, and Epilepsy

In some brain disorders, there's a problem with transporting glucose into the cells, which causes them to starve and die. Diseases that display a decreased glucose uptake into brain/nerve cells include:

- ALS/Lou Gehrig's disease
- Alzheimer's disease
- Autism (some forms)
- Down syndrome
- Duchenne muscular dystrophy
- Huntington's chorea
- Multiple sclerosis
- Parkinson's disease
- Type 1 and type 2 diabetes

Studies have revealed that neurons that can't use glucose can burn ketones. This means that ketones can provide the energy needed in these cells, potentially offering a therapeutic advantage in these brain disorders. Most studies have focused on the neuroprotective role of ketone bodies in patients with Alzheimer's disease, and a few studies show modest functional improvements in patients with Parkinson's disease.[7]

Keto for PCOS

Polycystic ovary syndrome is the most common endocrine disorder among women of reproductive age, affecting approximately 4 percent of women. PCOS is often associated with symptoms of excess testosterone: irregular or absent menses, extra body hair, and infertility. PCOS is also linked to medical abnormalities such as central obesity, insulin resistance, hyperinsulinemia, type 2 diabetes mellitus, and dyslipidemia.

Recent studies have shown that a low-carbohydrate, ketogenic diet can lead to weight loss and improvements in insulin resistance.[8]

Keto for Cancer

Research has shown that cancer cells rely on sugar for energy, a phenomenon termed "the Warburg effect." A keto diet can help prevent the growth of cancer cells, because it starves tumors of their primary energy source, glucose, while providing energy from fat for healthy cells.[9] Eliminating most carbohydrates and increasing ketone production creates a metabolic state similar to fasting, destroying cancer cells while preserving normal cells. Keto also inhibits insulin/IGF pathways and contains tumor growth and spread. Ongoing clinical trials are examining the potential of keto in cancer treatment, hoping to validate its effectiveness and safety in multiple types of cancer. By targeting cancer cells' metabolic weakness, ketogenic diets offer a promising complementary therapy to conventional cancer treatments, potentially improving patient outcomes.

When my client Kali Moynihan was 31 years old and pregnant with her first child, she was told that she had stage 4 cancer. She was given only a 20 percent chance of surviving five years, but after major surgery, she was determined not only to survive for her baby but also to truly heal and reclaim her life. I helped Kali achieve and maintain therapeutic ketosis, and within months her strength returned, her energy was better than before she had cancer, and she became deeply in tune with her body. Four years later, she has healed physically, emotionally, and spiritually. Her scans remain stable, and she continues to flex in and out of keto and fasting, supported by a low-glycemic lifestyle. Kali is living proof that when you trust your body and commit to a metabolic approach to healing, extraordinary things can happen.

Keto for Obesity

We've already established that being overweight is a symptom, not the actual problem. Obesity is an extreme symptom. Contrary to popular belief, genetics alone play a very small role here. When you eat more fat and protein, your body will produce wonderful chemicals called cholecystokinin (CCK), peptide YY, and leptin, which all prevent overconsumption. In addition, when you eat a very low-carbohydrate diet, a natural by-product will be lower insulin and blood sugar levels, which allow the body to tap into excess fat for fuel. Combine this with our intermittent-fasting strategies and you're on your way to an obesity-free life.

Keto for Cardiovascular Diseasez

The most common question/comment I receive on social media is about keto raising cholesterol. After guiding thousands of people through the keto lifestyle, I've observed that roughly 40 percent experience a rise in cholesterol levels—but that's not necessarily a bad thing. Most conventional doctors would view this as a harmful process; however, evidence from both experimental and clinical research has uncovered a protective role for ketones in cardiovascular disease. Although ketones may provide supplemental fuel for the energy-starved heart, they have also been shown to influence a variety of cellular processes, including gene transcription, inflammation and oxidative stress, endothelial function, cardiac remodeling, and cardiovascular risk factors.[10]

Keto for Longevity

The growing body of research on ketogenic diets points toward potential benefits for promoting longevity and combating age-related diseases. Three recent studies shed light on how ketogenic diets work at a molecular level, particularly focusing on how they tackle oxidative stress and regulate gene expression.

In one study from the National Library of Medicine, researchers investigated how ketones like beta-hydroxybutyrate (BHB) protect neurons from oxidative stress caused by glutamate excitotoxicity.[11] They found that ketones reduce the production of harmful reactive oxygen species in neurons by improving mitochondrial function. This could explain why ketogenic diets show promise in treating various neurological disorders.

An article published in *Graphical Review* delves into the multiple roles of BHB in managing stress responses and maintaining cellular balance. By inhibiting certain enzymes called histone deacetylases (HDACs), BHB increases the acetylation of histones, which are proteins involved in gene regulation.[12] This leads to changes in gene expression that enhance the body's ability to resist oxidative stress, which is particularly relevant in conditions like ischemia-reperfusion injury.

Another study by the National Library of Medicine sheds light on the potential of keto to extend lifespan and enhance health span in aging mice. Through an investigation using an iso-protein keto approach, the research uncovered significant benefits, including a reduction in midlife mortality without affecting maximum lifespan. An iso-protein approach means that protein intake is kept the same between comparison groups, while other variables—such as carbohydrates and fats—are adjusted. In this case, calories and protein were held constant, allowing researchers to isolate the effects of macronutrient composition and metabolic state (ketosis) rather than changes in protein quantity. Particularly noteworthy was the effectiveness of a cyclic keto diet, alternated weekly with a control diet to prevent obesity, in yielding these positive outcomes. The study also observed improvements in memory performance in older age and modest enhancements in overall health-span measures associated with keto. Gene expression analysis unveiled common downregulation of insulin, protein synthesis, and fatty-acid-synthesis pathways between a keto and a nonketogenic, high-fat diet. Notably, keto uniquely upregulated PPARα target genes consistently across various tissues, a pattern preserved in old age. This upregulation helps reduce inflammation and oxidative stress, supporting youthful, efficient metabolism even as you age.[13]

Lastly, a third study by the National Library of Medicine focused on how BHB acts as an HDAC inhibitor to suppress oxidative stress and activate genes that protect against it. They found that both fasting and ketogenic diets, which increase BHB levels, lead to higher histone acetylation and improved expression of genes involved in antioxidant defense.[14]

Together, these studies suggest that ketogenic diets, by increasing levels of beneficial ketones like BHB, could be a promising strategy for promoting longevity and reducing the risk of age-related diseases. By targeting oxidative stress and influencing gene expression, ketogenic diets offer potential avenues for improving overall health and lifespan. However, further research is needed to fully understand their long-term effects and mechanisms of action.

▲▼▲

You know *why* ketosis is good for your health—and better than traditional diets—but in the next chapter I'll explain exactly *how* ketosis works. You'll learn how to ease yourself into the Keto Flex lifestyle so that it's not a struggle, how to test your ketone levels, which blood tests will provide important information about your health, and how to ultimately measure your success.

CHAPTER FOUR

METABOLIC READINESS: SETTING THE STAGE FOR YOUR TRANSFORMATION

Like fasting, ketosis has a long history as a therapeutic tool. *Keto* may be a hot word in our cultural lexicon, but it's important to remember that it's a metabolic process, not a fad diet. If you do it properly, it can have lasting health benefits. In this chapter I'll explain more about how ketosis works and why it's crucial to ease into it rather than immediately going full throttle, which risks waking the primitive brain.

Think of this chapter as the foundation of everything you need to know before you begin the 45-day program. I'll introduce the four pillars of the Keto Flex Reset: Adapt, Fast, Phase, and Flex. I've intentionally designed these pillars so that your body can slowly adjust to the metabolic changes and feel good every step of the way. I'll also share the nine most important blood tests that will give you real, measurable data on your health. You'll learn how to test your ketone levels so that you know what to look for as you begin the reset in Chapter 5. Finally, I'll teach you the best ways to measure your success on the program (hint: They have nothing to do with the number on the scale).

WHAT IS KETOSIS?

Ketogenesis is the metabolic pathway that produces ketone bodies, which provide an alternative form of energy for the body. The term is based on *keto* (ketone body) and *genesis* (birth). Here's the bottom line in plain English: Ketones are a form of fuel made by your liver. Your liver produces ketones when your blood is low on glucose, which your body ordinarily uses for energy, or you don't have enough insulin in your bloodstream to turn sugar into glucose. Because you always need energy for your brain and muscles, your liver turns fat into ketones—a type of acid—and sends them into your bloodstream. Your brain, muscles, and other tissues can then use these ketones for fuel. Most organs and tissues can use ketone bodies as an alternative source of energy. During periods when glucose is not readily available, the brain uses them as a major source of energy. The heart typically uses fatty acids as its source of energy, but it can also use ketones.[1]

The goal of the Keto Flex lifestyle is to ensure your body flips the switch to fat burning and regularly enters in and out of a state of ketosis, where your blood contains a high concentration of ketones that your cells can use for energy. When ketones are produced faster than they can be used, they can be broken down into CO_2 and acetone. The acetone is removed by exhalation, which is why your breath smells sweet, like alcohol, during ketogenesis.

When you sharply cut your intake of carbohydrates, you'll experience lowered levels of circulating blood sugar (glucose) derived from those carbohydrates. In response, your body will look for energy elsewhere. It will start breaking down stored fat and changing it into those ketone bodies. Once you have ketones circulating in your blood, your cells will consume these ketone bodies to generate energy until you start eating carbohydrates again. Ketones can cross the blood-brain barrier and be used by the brain for fuel. Our hunter-gatherer ancestors, who endured long periods of quasi-starvation as they searched for game, burned their body fat, entering ketosis and using ketones to fuel their brains.

Scientists say the shift from using circulating glucose to breaking down stored fat as a source of energy usually begins over the course of two to four days of eating fewer than 20 to 50 grams of total carbohydrates per day. Everyone is different, and the process is highly individualized, so some people need a more restricted diet to start producing enough ketones.

Ketosis is good for many reasons (some of which we explored in the last chapter), but primarily because instead of relentlessly storing fat, your body can reclaim it and use it for energy, which is precisely why it's there in the first place. Your body designed its fat cells to serve as a backup energy supply, and ketosis takes advantage of the thousands of "free" calories locked in your cells in the form of fat. We say "free" because they cost you nothing. You paid for them long ago, in the form of the food you ate weeks, months, or even years ago. Ketosis removes this excess fat and puts it to good use. It's like your refrigerator and your freezer.

Your refrigerator is your short-term storage unit for food. Nothing stays in there very long; it contains the food you eat every day. But let's say you have an excess of food. What should you do with it? You store it in your freezer until you need to eat it. Well, over many millions of years, your body has been trained to be thrifty. It believes that since a food shortage could occur at any time—and painful experience has proved this to be true repeatedly—you need a backup supply of energy. If you had excess calories from a rice harvest or from killing a big wooly mammoth, then you needed to store them away for tomorrow. Your body does this in the form of fat just like you do this with a freezer full of food at home.

But what happens if you never eat the food in your freezer, because your refrigerator is always full of fresh food? And, because you're always cooking more than you need, you keep adding to that freezer? Then your freezer fills up. And because you're relentlessly thrifty, you buy another freezer. When that one is full, you buy another one. Eventually, you live in a house full of freezers, all full of food. The electricity bill is very high! If one day you emptied out your refrigerator and there was no food in it, what would you do? You'd open the freezer and use some of your stored food. If you kept doing this, a little bit at a time, eventually you could get rid of some of your freezers.

Sadly, the "buy more freezers" scenario has been playing out in Okinawa, the island group in Japan that for centuries was known for the longevity and good health of its people.

During the postwar era up until the year 2000, Okinawa had the longest life expectancy in all of Japan and one of the longest in the world. The local diet consisted of green and yellow vegetables, fish, relatively smaller amounts of rice compared to mainland Japan, pork, and soy and other legumes. The staple of the Okinawan diet was the Satsuma sweet potato. The traditional Okinawan diet had only 30 percent of the sugar and 15 percent of the grains of the average Japanese dietary intake, which itself was better than the aptly named standard American diet, or SAD.

The traditional Okinawan diet brought many benefits, including minimal weight gain with age, low body mass index (BMI) throughout life, and low risk from age-related diseases. The diet was also rich in ingredients that were said to possess anti-aging and antioxidant properties, such as turmeric. Like in many cultures, people in Okinawa believed in the healing power of food, which they regarded as medicine . . . and the reason for their longevity.

But the postwar era changed everything. Okinawa was occupied by US troops for 27 years, from the end of World War II to May 1972, and the American presence still looms large in the form of fast-food chains. In 1948, Blue Seal ice cream arrived, and the US company built a factory at Tengan military base to provide dairy products to the troops. The local population grew to love them. In 1963, American fast-food chain A&W introduced root beer, hamburgers, and curly fries to Okinawa. Now the island is crammed with franchise outlets like McDonald's, Burger King, KFC, MOS Burger, King Tacos, Subway, Mister Donut, and other purveyors of salt, sugar, and carbohydrates disguised as food. Not surprisingly, the life expectancy of young Okinawans, who never knew the local diet, has plummeted. Their digestive systems are taking in too many calories and storing the excess as fat . . . and the health problems are following right behind.

Today, the legendary lifespan of Okinawans is a thing of the past, and the residents are dying from Western diseases—heart attacks and diabetes—at the same rate as Americans.

The point is this: Eat a healthy diet. Keep your refrigerator half full, and when it gets empty, leverage the power of ketosis by going to the freezer, taking some of that free food energy, and enjoying it!

THE NOT-SO-NEW HISTORY OF KETO

Let's clear up one bit of misinformation about keto: It's not a diet; it's a metabolic process. It's nothing new—it's just nuanced. Its origins lie deep in human history, as every single one of our ancestors entered a state of ketosis, either unintentionally because food was scarce or intentionally for healing.

In ancient times, epilepsy and its scary seizures confounded natural philosophers, who attributed the disease to supernatural attacks from evil spirits. The legendary Greek physician Hippocrates discovered that somehow—he didn't know why—fasting was an effective therapy for combating epilepsy. As the centuries unfolded after Hippocrates, other physicians achieved the same results. They saw that the number and severity of epileptic seizures decreased if the patient fasted. There was a problem, though: Prolonged fasting is not a long-term solution to anything, because the outcome is death by starvation, which no one wants.

In 1911, worldwide interest in fasting to treat epilepsy was revived when two Paris doctors known as Guelpa and Marie published a paper in which they described how they could *mimic* the effects of fasting by using a special high-fat, low-carbohydrate diet. With their diet, which their patients could stay on indefinitely, they helped 20 people control their epilepsy, and they recorded the entire process in a report.[2]

In 1921, Dr. Russell Wilder, a pioneering researcher in diabetes and nutrition at the Mayo Clinic, developed a ketogenic therapy—the classic ketogenic diet—for the treatment of epilepsy. Like Guelpa and Marie, he realized that you could mimic the positive effects of fasting over many months and even years with a special high-fat, low-carb, low-protein diet. In Wilder's original formulation, "low protein" meant only about 6 to 8 percent of total calories, roughly 0.5–1 gram of protein per kilogram of body weight per day—a level designed not to build muscle but to mimic the fasting state and sustain deep, therapeutic ketosis for seizure control. The diet proved to be both perfectly healthy and effective against epilepsy. It was far more effective than phenobarbital and bromides, the only available anticonvulsant medications at the time. The ketogenic diet earned its place in the medical world as a therapy for pediatric epilepsy and was widely used until its popularity waned with the introduction of antiepileptic agents such as phenytoin (Dilantin).

In 1994, interest in the keto diet was revived when a little boy named Charlie Abrahams developed severe epilepsy that was unresponsive to medications, which gave him terrible side effects. After learning about the keto diet in a medical textbook, his parents took him to the Johns Hopkins Hospital in Baltimore, Maryland. Charlie began the diet, and within days his seizures stopped. He remained on the diet for five years. At last report, he lives on his own and remains seizure-free.

The family shared their story with the media, and thousands of letters poured in. Charlie's father, Jim Abrahams, was instrumental in bringing to the public the 1994 *Dateline* TV news magazine program "An Introduction to the Ketogenic Diet," featuring his friend, actress Meryl Streep. The same year he created the Charlie Foundation to help cure pediatric epilepsy. In 1997 he directed and produced *First Do No Harm*, a television movie starring Meryl Streep that was based on the true story of another child who also became seizure-free thanks to a ketogenic diet. This fostered increased worldwide interest and spurred further research that has proven the effectiveness of the diet as a treatment for epilepsy.

In many studies, the ketogenic diet has been shown to be particularly helpful for conditions such as infantile spasms, Rett syndrome, tuberous sclerosis complex, Dravet syndrome, Doose syndrome, and GLUT1 deficiency. Today, an epileptic seizure is defined as a transient symptom of abnormal excessive or synchronous firing of some or many of the brain's cells, or neurons. Why does fasting help control epilepsy? Science doesn't have the answer. It's like aspirin: No one knows precisely how it works, but it does.

In another twist to the story, while both intermittent fasting and the ketogenic diet reduce epileptic episodes in children, scientists believe they are not identical treatments and that they are effective through two different mechanisms.

WHY YOU SHOULD EASE INTO THE KETO FLEX LIFESTYLE

Any change to your diet that shocks your system is going to be hard to maintain. Recall the power of your reptilian or primal brain located in the basal ganglia. Not to mix too many animal metaphors, but this is the watchdog of your brain. It's always ready to detect the slightest threat to your safety and survival, including any drop in the amount of food you normally consume during the day. So, if you suddenly go on a "crash diet," it will alert your primal watchdog. You may be able to pat him on the head and placate him for a while, but eventually he'll start barking and creating a disturbance that you can't ignore. He'll make you so uncomfortable and miserable that to shut him up, you'll run to the kitchen or to McDonald's and pound down a few thousand calories.

There are mechanisms and receptors inside your body that give you signals when something is or isn't working. Small tweaks lead to giant peaks. You aren't competing against anyone else doing the Keto Flex lifestyle; your only competition is with yourself. What I teach my Fat Loss Academy students is simple: Your only competition is who you were yesterday. Every day is an opportunity to learn, improve, and get just a little bit better—to beat yesterday in every area of your health and life.

A common challenge arises when you make a self-imposed deadline for dropping a certain number of pounds. You see your high school reunion approaching, or a summer vacation that will require bathing suits, and you think, *OMG! I have to lose ten pounds in two weeks!*

Then you sign up for a fad diet or take weight-loss pills that promise to "melt away" your body fat. You hear testimonials from celebrities who lost weight quickly this way, probably because they were paid to do it. It's easy to believe you can slim down for the long term by using a fad diet, supplements, or pills. But these strategies are unsustainable. You can't take pills forever. You can't walk around all day feeling hungry and deprived because you're eating crappy "low-fat, low-calorie" food. That vigilant watchdog in your primal brain is barking his head off and driving you crazy. It's only a matter of time before you go back—with a vengeance—to your customary eating habits.

In the following chapters, I'll show you how you can ease yourself into the Keto Flex lifestyle with the 45-Day Keto Flex Reset, *one phase at a time*. Each phase is painless, and you should start the next phase only when you're comfortable.

Look at it this way: Unless you've been overweight since childhood, you've probably gained weight as an adult. The Centers for Disease Control and Prevention (CDC) reports that the average person typically puts on one to two pounds per year from early adulthood through middle age.[3] The CDC's numbers show the average man in his 20s weighs around 185 pounds. But by his 30s, he's closer to 200 pounds. The average woman's weight increases from about 162 to 170 pounds over the same period. So, let's say that like many Americans, you've gained 20 pounds over a period of 10 or 15 years. Why do you think it would be possible to drop those 20 pounds in even one year? That would require a massive effort, and that watchdog in your primal brain would be barking in your ear every step of the way. The odds of you giving up and putting the weight right back on again are extremely high.

You've probably heard the term "yo-yo dieting." It's a very real phenomenon. Every day, millions of Americans are looking for a new diet to try. Women are more concerned with weight loss than men (56.3 percent and 42.2 percent, respectively), and what is truly astonishing is that, according to various sources, the average dieter tries between 55 to 130 diets in their lifetime.

A 2020 survey conducted by Love Fresh Berries, a UK fresh-fruit trade organization, found that people don't stick to these fad diets for long. They usually abandon them after an average of only six days. More than half of respondents (52 percent) reported they were "really confused" about which of these fad diets were intended for a short-term period, and which were sustainable over long periods of time. The survey revealed that when it came to fad dieting, a lack of understanding and readily available information was a major obstacle. Overall, more than half were "baffled" regarding which foods should and shouldn't be cut out of their eating habits, and 20 percent of respondents said that they had no idea where to go for reliable dietary information.[4]

The Keto Flex Diet—or lifestyle, to be more accurate—is designed to be your road map to good nutrition for the rest of your life (barring, of course, the occasional slip). I always say, "It's never about the setback, it's about the get-back." The Keto Flex lifestyle is not carved in stone. It's a road map, not a set of commandments. It's not punitive—it's not designed to make you suffer. To the contrary, it should make you feel really good! The plan unfolds in a 45-Day Keto Flex Reset, which you take in easy succession, with four pillars:

1. **Adapt** (Days 1–7): Your body learns to switch from using sugar as its sole fuel source to occasionally using fat. You will effortlessly make the transition from burning sugar to burning fat (fat adaptation). No symptoms required!
2. **Fast** (Days 8–21): After you become fat adapted, you can move up to implement intermittent fasting so you can burn body fat and heal yourself. During this pillar, we practice various intermittent-fasting strategies as we build up your fasting muscle.
3. **Phase** (Days 22–45): Now you're ready to help your cells use fat as their only fuel source for a designated period of time. We practice the carnivore diet and phase out all carbohydrates and antinutrients. You will experience incredible digestive and brain health benefits here.
4. **Flex** (Day 46 and Beyond): This is where you develop the flexibility to intentionally move in and out of ketosis. The most common challenge with an ordinary keto diet is inherent to the diet. Many people who try a keto diet can't stick to it, or they have cravings, or they find the longer they stick with it, the more challenging it becomes to keep the weight off. As you'll discover, this flex approach is the differentiator. What I will show you in Pillar 4 is that a long-term keto diet can cause weight gain and hormone imbalance, and my Keto Flex approach prevents this and keeps you on the path to your ideal weight and perfect health. You will learn why women should follow keto differently than men as well as a specific protocol for you to achieve long-term results.

NINE IMPORTANT BLOOD TESTS

Don't guess, test! The more data you have, the more metrics you can analyze for progress and necessary tweaks. I will share the nine blood tests I recommend having before you start my 45-Day Keto Flex Reset. (Then you can test again after the reset to see how much your markers have improved.) Not only will I share the blood tests with you, but I will also explain what they mean and the optimal numbers to aim for, because the reference ranges on your lab report are not the same as the ideal healthy ranges. Lab companies such as Labcorp, Quest, and many others are factoring in your country's entire population who have done these labs before. We live in a sick world of unhealthy people, so why would we aim to be the average of unhealthy people? Instead, I encourage you to aim for the functional reference range. Functional medicine lab ranges are usually much narrower than standard lab ranges. They're labeled "optimal lab values," meaning anything outside of those optimal values can show patterns and markers that spot trends toward disease. When I give you the suggested reference ranges to hit with the following labs, these are functional medicine lab ranges.

1. Hemoglobin A1C

How gummed up with sugar are your blood cells? Hemoglobin A1C (HbA1c) measures your average blood sugar from the past three months. Hemoglobin A is a protein used by your red blood cells to carry oxygen to your tissues. The higher your blood sugar, the more glucose sticks to the hemoglobin A1c protein. This blood test measures how much glucose is stuck to the hemoglobin protein. Test your hemoglobin A1C to learn your average blood sugar. You can request this test from your doctor or do an A1C test kit in the comfort of your own home.

A 2020 study estimated that for both type 1 and type 2 diabetes, each year with an HbA1c greater than 7.5 percent is associated with a loss of roughly 100 days of life expectancy. I did the math for you: This means if your HbA1c levels are >7.5 percent for 15 years, you lose four years off your lifespan.[5] Linking blood sugar control to mortality has the potential to encourage us to embrace and adhere to a healthier lifestyle.

A "normal" A1C level is below 5.7 percent, a level of 5.7–6.4 percent indicates prediabetes, and a level of 6.5 percent or more indicates diabetes. Within the 5.7–6.4 percent prediabetes range, the higher your A1C, the greater your risk is for developing type 2 diabetes.

The functional medicine range of A1C is 5.2 percent or lower.

2. C-Peptide

C-peptide is a substance created when insulin is produced and released into the body. The C-peptide test reflects how much insulin your pancreas is producing, rather than measuring insulin directly. The pancreas makes insulin, but not directly. The beta cells in the pancreas first produce a protein called proinsulin. Each proinsulin breaks down to one molecule of insulin and one molecule of C-peptide. Both are released when blood sugar levels become high.

The more your beta cells get stimulated for insulin production, the faster you gain weight and create inflammation. While moderate levels lower inflammation, even slightly higher levels have been linked to insulin resistance, metabolic syndrome, heart disease, and cancer. C-peptide can give you a good idea if you've been overworking your beta cells.

Levels below 0.6 ng/mL (0.2 nmol/L) are a sign of possible beta cell failure and type 1 diabetes. High C-peptide levels indicate that the body is producing too much insulin.

The functional medicine range for C-peptide is 0.8–3.8 ng/mL.

3. Fasting Insulin

This test is a great complement to the C-peptide test. Testing your insulin can reveal hidden problems in the way your body controls your blood sugar years before they escalate to more serious issues, such as diabetes. In many cases, your blood sugar levels might not change for 10-plus years—meanwhile, you're getting closer each day to developing diabetes. This is because insulin is working so hard to keep those sugar levels "normal." After a period, insulin can't keep up with the demand. At this point, blood sugars start to rise, and a diagnosis of prediabetes or diabetes is made. A fasting insulin test allows you to see if you are insulin resistant or on the road to insulin resistance.

The standard reference range for fasting insulin is less than 25 uIU/mL.

The functional medicine range for fasting insulin is 3–6 uIU/mL.

4. 25-Hydroxy Vitamin D

Vitamin D is a fat-soluble vitamin (and hormone) the body needs to build and maintain strong bones. It helps absorb calcium in the gut, keeping calcium and phosphorus in balance to mineralize bones. Vitamin D also helps support immune balance. Most people are deficient in vitamin D.

Symptoms of vitamin D deficiency may include:

- Fatigue
- Not sleeping well
- Bone pain or achiness
- Depression or feelings of sadness
- Hair loss
- Muscle weakness
- Loss of appetite
- Getting sick more easily
- Pale skin

Is the solution taking vitamin D supplements? Not really. I'm not opposed to taking a fat-soluble complex supplement, but until you lower insulin, you won't be able to change your vitamin D numbers for the better. High insulin levels block the production of vitamin D! You can take all the vitamin D in the world and get sunshine every day, but you won't optimize your vitamin D levels until you optimize insulin. The great news for you is that this book will teach you how to do this.

The standard reference range on your lab report is typically 30–80 ng/mL.

The functional medicine range for vitamin D is 60–80 ng/mL.

5. Homocysteine

Homocysteine is an amino acid. High homocysteine has been linked to many health problems, including heart disease, dementia, and Alzheimer's. When homocysteine can't be converted to other compounds, it builds up in the body and may cause damage. B vitamins play an important role in this balance. Vitamins B_6, B_{12}, and folate work together to recycle homocysteine back into methionine, a process essential for DNA repair, detoxification, and brain health. When these nutrients are deficient, homocysteine can rise, increasing the risk for inflammation, cardiovascular disease, and cognitive decline. The Keto Flex approach naturally supports healthy homocysteine levels because it emphasizes nutrient-dense foods like pastured eggs, wild-caught fish, grass-fed meats, and leafy greens—all rich in these critical B vitamins. By improving methylation, lowering inflammation, and balancing insulin, Keto Flex helps restore the biochemical pathways that keep homocysteine in check and protect your heart, brain, and mitochondria.

The standard reference range for homocysteine is below 14.5 umol/L.

The functional medicine range for homocysteine is 5–7 umol/L.

6. High-Sensitivity C-Reactive Protein

This protein is an important marker of systemic inflammation. While C-reactive protein helps you fight infections, it's also a marker of low-grade inflammation and a predictor of your heart disease risk. People with higher hs-CRP values have a more elevated risk of cardiovascular disease, and those with lower values have less risk.

The standard reference range for hs-CRP is 0–3.0 mg/L.

The functional medicine range for hs-CRP is 0.5 mg/L or below.

7. High-Density Lipoprotein Count (HDL-C)

I often get asked about cholesterol, and the remaining blood tests are the true markers for heart disease risk (not total cholesterol, which is meaningless). Total cholesterol simply adds together HDL ("good"), LDL ("bad"), and very-low-density lipoprotein (VLDL) particles without telling you anything about their size, density, or function. A high total number could actually be healthy if it's driven by protective HDL or large, fluffy LDL particles that don't oxidize easily. What truly matters is insulin resistance, inflammation, and particle oxidation—because it's the damaged LDL particles, not cholesterol itself, that contribute to plaque formation. In other words, cholesterol is the fireman at the scene, not the arsonist—it's there to repair, not to destroy. HDL is often referred to as the "good" cholesterol because it helps remove the "bad" cholesterol and is required for many vital processes within the body. Having high levels of HDL cholesterol has been shown to decrease your risk for heart disease.

Cholesterol transported by HDL is known as "good" cholesterol because it's being removed from artery walls, which helps prevent, reduce, and even reverse the hardening of the arteries (atherosclerosis) and heart disease.[6]

HDL also plays a role in reducing oxidative stress and inflammation, improving cell and immune function, enhancing insulin sensitivity, and possibly protecting against neurodegenerative disorders.[7]

The standard reference range for HDL for men is 35–65 mg/dl and for women is 35–80 mg/dl.

The functional reference range for HDL for both men and women is 60–90 mg/dl.

8. Triglycerides

Triglycerides are a type of fat that can either be stored in fat tissue or used for energy. For example, the body can release stored fats into the bloodstream as fatty acids when you don't eat for a prolonged time. These fatty acids travel back to the liver, which transforms them into triglyceride-containing, very-low-density lipoproteins that are returned into the blood. On the other hand, your body stores more triglycerides when you overeat or have an unhealthy diet, such as the good ol' standard American diet. High levels of triglycerides can increase your risk of obesity, heart disease, diabetes, and other chronic health conditions.

The standard reference range for triglycerides is below 150 mg/dL.

The functional medicine range for triglycerides is below 90 mg/dL.

9. Triglycerides-to-HDL Ratio

Your triglycerides-to-HDL ratio (TG:HDL) helps offer a lifelong metric for your health. TG:HDL is one of the criteria for the diagnosis of metabolic syndrome, which was briefly known as Reaven syndrome, named after Gerald Reaven, MD, of Stanford University. He and his colleagues around the world pioneered much of the research on the TG:HDL ratio that indicates cardiovascular risk. It's a strong marker of lifestyle factors—your TG:HDL ratio offers a way to see whether you have a metabolism that naturally has cardiac protection or whether you need to earn it.

To calculate your TG:HDL ratio, you simply take your total triglycerides and divide this by your total HDL.

The standard reference range for TG:HDL is below 3.5.

The functional medicine range for TG:HDL is below 1.5.

HOW TO TEST YOUR KETONE LEVELS

There are three different methods for testing your ketone levels: urine, breath, and blood. Urine testing is helpful only in the beginning stages of fat adaptation, when your body is still learning how to use the ketones you're creating. During this time, a good portion of the ketone bodies' acetoacetate you produce will get filtered out through your urine. This can give insight into whether your body is producing ketones. However, over time, your body will become more adapted, and the number of ketones lost in your urine will decrease.

Breath testing is a valid way to test the ketone body's acetone, and it's much less invasive than blood testing—but it may be less accurate. I have recently discovered an accurate breath ketone meter from KetoAir.

The most common way to test ketones is with blood. I personally use the Keto-Mojo device that tests for BHB in the blood. You can purchase your Keto-Mojo device over at benazadi.com/ketomojo. The unit of measurement is the millimole. A mole is an amount of a substance that contains a large number (6 followed by 23 zeros) of molecules or atoms. Abbreviated *mmol*, a millimole is one-thousandth of a mole. It's measured per liter of blood, as in 1.0 mmol/L.

If your ketogenic goal is weight loss, then 0.5 mmol/L to 0.8 mmol/L is a good starting point. From there, aim for "optimal ketosis," which is when your ketone levels are between 0.8 mmol/L to 3.0 mmol/L. This is perfectly healthy and puts you in fat-burning mode. People using the ketogenic diet for its therapeutic benefits for medical conditions such as epilepsy, cancer, or endocrine and metabolic disorders might aim for much higher ketone levels, in the 3.0 mmol/L–to–5.0 mmol/L range. Those who are fasting or consuming a much higher fat-to-protein ratio can post levels in the range of 3.0 mmol/L to 8.0 mmol/L, but you don't need to aim that high. The optimal ketosis range is called "optimal" for a reason, and it's ideal for weight loss and general health purposes.

In the Keto Flex Reset, we do not chase ketones. We chase *results*.

Can you have too many ketones in your blood? Yes. Just like you can have too much sugar in your blood (hyperglycemia), you can have too many ketones, a condition called *ketoacidosis*. It's most often associated with type 1 diabetes and called *diabetic ketoacidosis*. Signs of diabetic ketoacidosis include excessive thirst, frequent urination, nausea, vomiting, abdominal pain, shortness of breath, fruity-scented breath, and confusion. Among nondiabetic people, with moderate and controlled fasting, ketoacidosis is usually not a problem.

MEASURING YOUR KETO SUCCESS

Keto is not to be used for quick weight loss. Will you lose weight with keto if this is your goal? Absolutely. But this happens because you're becoming healthier. The great news is that the weight stays off!

Throw away your bathroom scale! Why do I say this? Isn't measuring your weight important? As a part of your overall health, your weight is important. But looking at the scale and then saying, "I need to lose weight because then I'll be healthier" is putting the cart before the horse. It's "backasswards," as they say. It's the opposite of what you want to do. If you focus only on losing weight, you will be miserable, and you'll probably fail. Here's a question worth pondering: Do you know why the weight-loss industry in America is worth 2.6 billion dollars? It's because diet programs, where you enroll and eat the food they sell to you, have millions of *repeat customers*. They're repeat customers because traditional dieting, where the goal is to lose weight, fails. *It fails over and over again*. Sure, you may lose weight on a diet, but statistics prove that most people just gain back the pounds, so then they need to go back on a diet. It's called "yo-yo dieting" for a good reason.

The reasons for yo-yo dieting are varied but often include embarking upon a calorie-restricted diet that's too extreme and focused on the wrong foods. At first, the dieter experiences elation at the thought of weight loss and pride in their rejection of food. However, over time, the painful limits imposed by unnatural diets can cause depression or fatigue, making the diet impossible to sustain. The dieter inevitably reverts to their old eating habits, but now with the added psychological burden of having failed to lose weight by a restrictive diet.

In contrast, the Keto Flex lifestyle is focused on improving your *health*, beginning with your trillions of individual cells. Many people report a feeling of freedom—the opposite of the restrictive feeling of hallmark traditional diets. That's because Keto Flex doesn't fight your biology—it works with it. When you lower carbs and sugar, your body shifts from glucose dependency to fat adaptation, and healthy fats and proteins naturally satisfy your hunger hormones. Instead of triggering cravings and blood sugar crashes that activate the primal "food-seeking" part of your brain, you feel calm, clear, and in control. You're not relying on willpower—you're rewiring your metabolism to crave freedom, not food. You'll feel the difference in your energy level, your overall happiness, and the tone of your body. Will you lose weight? As you burn fat for energy, yes, you will. But that just goes along with the idea that if you correct an underlying condition, the symptoms—in this case, excess body fat—will take care of themselves.

I want you to focus on non-scale victories (NSVs). This is how you will get accurate data on whether this is working for you. Non-scale victories include, but are not limited to, improvements in the following:

- How your clothes fit
- Monthly photos
- Body-fat percentage
- Energy levels
- Skin health
- Gut health
- Confidence
- Mental health

I encourage you to step away from the scale and pay close attention to these NSVs. Give yourself 45 days of following the 45-Day Keto Flex Reset and then you can step on the scale. You will be pleasantly surprised by the results.

I challenge you to take "before" photos of yourself right now. No one needs to see them but you. Take front-facing photos, side-facing photos, and photos of your back. After 45 days, retake these photos and compare them. They will give you visual proof of your health transformation.

▲▼▲

We've laid the groundwork so you know what to expect, how to measure your ketones, and you've had all of your blood tests. You're ready to start your 45-day Keto Flex Reset! In the next chapter, you'll begin Pillar 1: Adapt. I'll show you not only which foods to avoid and why but also which ones to add, including the best choices for fats and protein. And I'll also give you some easy-to-follow meal plans to make the transition as smooth as possible.

CHAPTER FIVE

THE 45-DAY KETO FLEX RESET

Welcome to your 45-Day Keto Flex Reset! In the last chapters, we explored the science and history of keto as well as some of the logistics about testing. But if you really want *results*, you need to take *action*, and in this chapter we'll start to implement this powerful metabolic tool. We're going to explore two equally important components of the Keto Flex lifestyle: *what* you eat and *when* you eat it. You can't pay attention to one without paying attention to the other.

The goal of this reset is to help you achieve metabolic flexibility via ketosis and intermittent fasting. The 45-Day Keto Flex Reset has four essential pillars:

1. **Adapt:** teaching your metabolism to burn fat instead of sugar to provide your body with a cleaner energy source
2. **Fast:** implementing fasting strategies to build up your metabolic machinery further
3. **Phase:** resetting your digestive system by removing the most common foods that irritate your gut
4. **Flex:** working with your hormones to flex in and out of ketosis, based on your gender, age, and health status

These ancient healing strategies have stood the test of time, and this reset will help you integrate the Keto Flex concepts into your life much quicker. It's the exact blueprint I've used on thousands of people around the world. In this chapter you'll begin the first pillar (Adapt), where you'll wean off carbohydrates and eliminate harmful oils and chemicals and replace them with healthy fats and proteins.

WHO IS THIS RESET FOR?

Keto Flex is for everyone! Burning fat is your primal birthright. Although there are numerous health benefits to this reset (many of which we explored in Chapter 3), here are some of the symptoms and conditions that it helps the most:

- Accelerated aging
- Autoimmune conditions
- Brain fog
- Cardiovascular conditions
- Diabetes and prediabetes
- Gut dysbiosis (leaky gut)
- Hair loss
- Hormonal cancers
- Infertility challenges
- Insulin resistance
- Lack of motivation
- Low energy
- Memory problems
- Menopause symptoms
- Mood disorders such as anxiety and depression
- PCOS
- Thyroid conditions
- Weight-loss resistance

Of course, it's best to work with your doctor and inform them of your new Keto Flex lifestyle when you're about to start.

WHEN TO START YOUR RESET

Be sure to look at your social calendar before starting the reset. Do you have any weddings, vacations, or events coming up? This can potentially derail your progress. Peer pressure can cause most people to get off track, so I suggest starting this reset when you know your next 45 days are clear of any occasions that might take you off course. The great news is that once you get the hang of this reset, you'll see that the Keto Flex lifestyle fits into the busiest of lives.

Before You Start

As you embark on this life-changing reset, it's important to ask yourself why you're doing this. Your real *why* is usually layers behind what you think it is. For example, most people say their why is to lose 50 pounds. When I ask them why that's their reason, they may say something like, "I want to feel lighter." I then ask them again, "Why?" Then they may say, "I want to have more energy for my children. Right now, I'm exhausted from spending time with them." This is the *real* reason. When the why is strong, the how becomes easier.

PILLAR 1: ADAPT TO FAT BURNING

I call the first pillar *Adapt* because the goal is getting you fat adapted, and I've carefully designed your entry into the Keto Flex lifestyle to be pleasant. The first seven days are all about getting you to burn fat instead of sugar without experiencing any symptoms as you make this transition to the great land of ketosis. If you need more time, that's fine! We don't want to arouse the ire of your primal-brain watchdog—we respect him, know his power, and want to keep him peacefully sleeping. Just keep at it. You'll find that the fewer carbs and sugars you eat, the less of them you'll want. Even if you cut your carbs in half, you'll be happier and healthier.

First, let's review how your body processes food into energy. When you eat food—a mix of carbs, protein, and fat—your digestive system converts molecules from the carbs and proteins into molecules of glucose, which are transferred into your bloodstream and raise your blood sugar level. As blood glucose levels rise, the pancreas secretes insulin. This hormone performs several key functions: It acts as a transporter, carrying glucose to the cells in the body, where it's used as an energy source. When the blood glucose enters liver cells, the insulin stimulates the action of several enzymes, including glycogen synthase (for the conversion of glucose into glycogen). While both insulin and glucose remain plentiful, glucose molecules are added to the clumps of glycogen.

Additionally, when there is excess glucose in the bloodstream, known as *hyperglycemia*, insulin encourages the storage of glucose as glycogen in the liver, muscle, and fat cells. These stores can then be used later, when energy requirements are higher or when food is scarce, such as when you're fasting. As a result, there's less insulin in the bloodstream, and normal blood glucose levels are restored. In simplified form, the "glucose chain" goes like this: You eat food, which releases glucose into the bloodstream. The glucose travels to the liver, where it's combined with insulin to make glycogen, which can be stored.

Think of glycogen as your sugar reserves. Do you remember the refrigerator-versus-freezer analogy earlier in the book? Here's a reminder: I'm going to compare these sugar reserves to the refrigerator in your kitchen. It's easy access—you just open the door and take out fresh food, ready to eat. Your fat stores are more difficult to get to—they're like the freezer in your basement. The food in your freezer is more difficult to access—you have to go downstairs, retrieve the frozen food, and then thaw it out.

Recall we talked about being a "fat burner" versus a "sugar burner." Here's a handy equation to remember:

high insulin levels = sugar burner
low insulin levels = fat burner

What's fascinating is that fat is the only type of food that has almost no effect on insulin. You can eat all the fat you want, and it will not give you the insulin spikes that carbs do. This is why the first step in your 45-Day Keto Flex Reset is to gradually remove most of the carbohydrates in your diet and replace them with healthy fats and protein.

INSULIN RESISTANCE AND DIABETES

As a side note, in type 2 diabetes, which is at near-epidemic levels in the industrialized world, the muscle, fat, and liver cells build *insulin resistance*. They don't allow insulin to carry the glucose into the cell, which is bad, because every cell needs glucose to survive. I know, it sounds weird that your cells would refuse to accept a delivery of groceries, but that's what happens. In response, the pancreas churns out more insulin. For a while, this strategy works, and your blood sugar levels remain normal. But over time, your pancreas can't keep up, and your blood sugar levels rise until you have prediabetes.

YOUR EATING PATTERN FOR THE FIRST 7 DAYS

We're going to keep this simple. Don't worry about counting calories or measuring your serving sizes; eat until full. Yes—really! The human body doesn't have any mechanisms for counting calories, so why are so many people meticulously tracking every calorie they consume? You're not a calculator. You're not a math equation. You're a complex chemistry lab with sophisticated internal checks and balances.

The first step is to eat *three meals* per day. If you're the average person who works during the day, you'll probably follow a schedule like this: breakfast at 7 A.M., lunch at 1 P.M. (six hours later), and dinner at 7 P.M. (six hours later). If you tend to eat a later breakfast or earlier dinner, that's fine. You don't need to have exactly six hours between each meal—the primary goal is to stick to three meals per day, with no snacking in between. Then you have 12 hours until breakfast the next day. Many people get nervous when they think about going 12 hours with no food, but trust me, that's the way your digestive system was designed. Those 12 hours are important to clear out your stomach, lower your insulin levels, and stabilize your blood sugar. You're giving your body a break from producing insulin every time you eat, which can prevent or reverse insulin resistance. And I'll bet that when you wake up in the morning, you won't feel ravenous; you'll feel normal and clearheaded, ready to enjoy the day.

Carbohydrate Quantities

Most people can enter into ketosis by limiting their total carbohydrates to 50 grams per day, although longtime sugar burners may need to be more restrictive. I don't recommend dropping your carbohydrates below 50 total grams too soon, because when you aggressively lower your carbohydrates, it can lead to symptoms that may make you want to quit the reset. Instead, I suggest a gradual approach.

While keeping your eating schedule to three meals per day, you will gradually decrease your carbohydrates. Please note, I'm basing this off the average person who consumes 300 grams or more of carbohydrates per day. With many Americans consuming this many carbohydrates per day, it's no surprise why Harvard predicts that by the year 2030, half of the United States population will be classified as obese.[1] Feel free to customize this approach depending on how many carbohydrates you are currently consuming. Here's what this looks like:

Day 1: 250 grams of total carbohydrates per day
Day 2: 150 grams of total carbohydrates per day
Day 3: 100 grams of total carbohydrates per day
Day 4: 75 grams of total carbohydrates per day
Day 5: 50 grams or less of total carbohydrates per day
Day 6: Ketosis unlocked! Let the metabolic magic begin.

You can use an app like Cronometer to keep track of your carbohydrates,* and make sure you are tracking total carbohydrates instead of net carbohydrates. Visit cronometer.com/ketokamp to download this free app. Total carbs include all the carbohydrates in a food—fiber, sugar alcohols, and starches—while net carbs subtract the fiber and sometimes sugar alcohols, assuming they have little impact on blood sugar. I prefer tracking total carbs because it keeps things transparent and prevents people from underestimating their intake, which often stalls fat loss and ketosis. If you're having difficulty getting into ketosis, see Chapter 10 for more information and troubleshooting tips.

Foods to Avoid

As you begin your reset, it's important to know which foods to avoid. And I'm not just talking about carbs. There are many foods that may technically help you achieve ketosis, but that doesn't mean those foods are good for you, especially at the cellular level.

Vegetable Oils and Other Inflammatory Fats

Not every fat is a good fat. There are bad, rancid fats that wreak havoc in our body. Vegetable oils are bad fats because they cause inflammation in our cells, which interferes with the communication from our hormones, nutrients, and oxygen. It becomes harder for nutrients and hormones to enter our cells and for toxins to leave our cells.

* You can find it at www.cronometer.com/ketokamp.

The harmful oils you want to avoid are:

- Canola oil (also called rapeseed oil)
- Corn oil
- Cottonseed oil
- Fish oil (extracted fish oil oxidizes, while whole fish stays fresh and protected)
- Grapeseed oil
- Hydrogenated oil
- Refined palm oil
- Refined peanut oil
- Rice bran oil
- Safflower oil
- Soybean oil
- Sunflower oil

Pro tip: When at restaurants, tell your server that you're allergic to the above oils and ask them to use a healthier alternative. I created a vegetable oil allergy card that you can print out and take with you. Download it for free by heading to seedoilcard.com.

Can you remove damaged fats such as vegetable oils from your cells? Yes, you can. Fasting is a great way to help your body remove them faster through the process of autophagy, mitophagy, apoptosis, and stem-cell production.

Chemicals

You also want to avoid a group of foods that are filled with chemicals. Many of these chemicals create inflammation inside your body, which ultimately will make your keto experience really hard. These chemicals are often referred to as *obesogens*. Many of them can spike both glucose and insulin and can stimulate the hunger centers in your brain. This makes the keto lifestyle more difficult to sustain. They are in many keto products, so make sure you read the label.

Common synthetic ingredients to avoid:

- Acesulfame potassium
- Artificial colors and flavorings
- Aspartame
- NutraSweet
- Red or blue dyes
- Saccharin
- Sucralose

Other Tricky Foods

To give you a head start with resetting your fat-burning hormones, I also recommend you remove the following foods from your diet, at least for the duration of this 45-Day Keto Flex Reset. I've seen this significantly reduce inflammation inside the body, which leads to better results:

- Almonds (high in oxalates, oxalates are plant defense chemicals that can bind minerals and irritate tissues in some people; replace with macadamia nuts, walnuts, pecans, and pili nuts)
- Corn (typically GMO)
- Pasteurized cow dairy (replace with raw cow dairy or sheep/goat dairy)
- Legumes (including peanuts and chickpeas)
- Nightshades (tomatoes, potatoes, goji berries, peppers, eggplant)
- Soy (organic fermented soy such as natto and tempeh are fine)
- Spinach and kale (high in oxalates; replace with arugula and broccoli)

While many consider these "keto friendly" foods, you will accelerate your results by removing them from your diet.

Foods to Add

It's not just important to remove some of the harmful foods that you've been consuming throughout your lifetime; you also need to know which foods to incorporate during your reset for the best results. The goal is to prevent unwanted symptoms such as cravings. The best way to stop these cravings is to stabilize your blood sugar and kill the hunger hormone ghrelin. This can be accomplished by adding more good fats and protein to your diet.

Good Fats: The 2/2/2/2 Rule

For your first seven days, as you lower carbohydrates, I recommend you follow the 2/2/2/2 rule, which will help your body utilize fatty acids for fuel instead of glucose. This rule makes the transition much smoother. As you lower total carbohydrates the first week of your reset, the goal is to train your body to switch fuel sources over to fat. You can give your innate intelligence an assist here by adding in healthy fats, in abundance.* For the first seven days of phase 1, Adapt, consume the following:

- 2 tablespoons of grass-fed butter or grass-fed ghee
- 2 tablespoons of coconut oil or MCT oil
- 2 tablespoons of beef tallow, avocado oil, or extra-virgin olive oil
- 2 teaspoons of sea salt

When I introduce this rule, people often ask, "How do I get all of these fats in one sitting?" You don't—you spread them out between all your meals. For example, you would use them for cooking oils, salad dressings, dips, and/or to include with your coffee or tea. If you find you're having loose stools from following the 2/2/2/2 rule, cut it in half (we'll call it the 1/1/1/1 rule).

You may be wondering why I included sea salt in the 2/2/2/2 rule. This is because of something people refer to as the "keto flu" (more on this in Chapter 10). As your body adjusts to any change of diet—especially one that is moving you toward better health—there may be some initial side effects. The most common and relatively minor short-term side effects of beginning the Keto Flex lifestyle may include nausea, vomiting, headache, fatigue, dizziness, insomnia, difficulty in exercise tolerance, and constipation. These "keto flu" symptoms can more accurately be described as carbohydrate-withdrawal symptoms. They usually resolve in a few days to a few weeks. Not all people will exhibit these symptoms when going through the diet transition period. Some can switch to a keto diet with little to no side effects.

What causes the keto flu? It's really quite simple. Carbohydrates are stored in the body with water. When you lower your carb intake, your

* Credit goes to my mentor, Dr. Daniel Pompa, for this one.

body initially responds by excreting more water and retaining less. As you lose water, you may quickly gain a "lean" look. Fewer carbs means less insulin release, causing the kidneys to release more sodium. This loss of sodium impacts the balance of other key electrolytes, including potassium and magnesium. These are minerals that carry an electrical charge. Vital for health and survival, they spark cell function throughout the body, support hydration, and help the body produce energy. As carb intake decreases and electrolytes are increasingly excreted from the body in urine, imbalances of these electrolytes trigger the keto flu symptoms.[2]

Ensuring adequate fluid and electrolyte intake can help counter some of these symptoms. Consuming two teaspoons of sea salt per day, throughout the day, should prevent them from occurring.

Once ketosis is achieved by registering 0.5 or higher on your Keto-Mojo, you can stop the 2/2/2/2 rule, because keto is not about eating high fat, especially when you want to burn body fat. We'll focus on the value of protein at this point.

THE BEST FATS

For cooking at high temperatures (375°F or higher), you can use:

- Butter
- Ghee
- Beef tallow
- Duck fat
- Lard (nonhydrogenated from pastured pigs)
- Coconut oil

For salad dressings, dips, and medium to low-heat cooking:

- Avocado oil
- Extra-virgin olive oil

Protein

Many people who first learn about keto assume that it's antiprotein, or that protein is bad for you. They also cite many other objections to eating protein, all of which are easily dismantled. They believe that keto is a high-fat-only diet. This isn't true. Most keto gurus will tell you that too much protein will kick you out of ketosis, but I haven't seen this to be the case. Excess amino acids from digested protein must be oxidized as fuel or converted into other storage products. The excess ingested protein can, through the process of gluconeogenesis, produce glucose. This would mean that 100 grams of protein could produce about 50 grams of glucose. This should not kick you out of ketosis, since the glucose produced will refill your glycogen stores (sugar reserves) found in your liver and skeletal muscle.

Protein is arguably the most important macronutrient. Amino acids are crucial for building healthy bodies. How much protein should you have on keto? For the first seven days, your focus is on consuming enough fat via the 2/2/2/2 rule and getting your total carbohydrates below 50 grams by Day 7, so we won't focus on specific grams. Simply consume as much protein as you wish with your meals in the form of eggs, chicken, fish, or beef to help you feel full. In Pillar 2, we start prioritizing protein, and I'll outline how much protein to hit each day.

Protein is required for fat burning. *Essentials of Biochemistry* reveals, "Carnitine, an amino acid from protein, is essential for fat-burning. A deficiency in this protein automatically means a deficiency in fat-burning capability."

Another benefit of a Keto Flex approach emphasizing animal protein is the feeling of satiety. When you eat dietary protein, it activates the following chemicals to help you feel full:

- Cholecystokinin
- Leptin
- Glucagon-like peptide (GLP-1)
- Peptide YY

These are processes that signal your brain to put down the fork. For example, if you feast on a 20-ounce rib eye steak, and someone offers you their rib eye steak, chances are you'd feel too satisfied and full to eat another steak. If the same person offered you their ice cream, or cookie, after you'd eaten your own ice cream, chances are you'd have room to eat more. Why? Because carbohydrates do not activate the same signals, which is why it's so much easier to overeat carbs than it is protein.

Some people worry that too much protein will create kidney issues. According to the textbook *Basic Medical Biochemistry*, "Glutamine (an amino acid from protein) removes all of the ammonia, a normal by-product of protein metabolism, from your bloodstream."[3] And Professor Brian Peskin's book *The 24-Hour Diet* states, "Protein on its own can't enter the kidney. It needs a lot of sugar to carry it in. It is the carbohydrates that cause kidney damage."[4] So, as you can see, protein will not harm your kidneys. (That said, if you have any kidney issues—or any health issues—I always recommend speaking to your doctor before you begin any dietary changes.)

Healthy proteins to add:

- Grass-fed-and-finished beef and lamb
- Pastured turkey and chicken
- Bison
- Pastured pork
- Pastured eggs
- Charcuterie meats like salami and prosciutto
- Sardines
- Salmon
- Anchovies
- Herring
- Mackerel

KETO-APPROVED CLEAN SWEETENERS

- Erythritol
- Xylitol
- Swerve
- Pure stevia
- Monk fruit
- Allulose

EXAMPLE KETO MEAL PLAN

Breakfast

Option 1	5 runny, sunny-side-up eggs with 1/2 avocado and 2 cups of arugula, cooked in grass-fed butter. Sprinkle 2 tablespoons of nutritional yeast.
Option 2	Fatty (keto) smoothie consisting of 3/4 cup of full-fat coconut milk, 1/4 cup of water, 1/2 avocado, 2 full scoops of grass-fed collagen protein powder, 2 tablespoons of organic raw walnut butter, and ice. (Skip the toast or muffin!)

Lunch

Option 1	Fatty salad with 2 to 4 cups of arugula, 2 tablespoons of extra-virgin olive oil, a handful of raw macadamia nuts, sea salt, and black pepper. For protein, add an 8-ounce piece of wild salmon or grass-fed beef.
Option 2	Spaghetti squash noodles with 8 ounces of sliced free-range chicken and a handful of raw macadamia nuts. Drizzle with extra-virgin olive oil.

Dinner

Option 1	1 cup of steamed brussels sprouts with a sprinkle of sea salt and 1 tablespoon of melted butter on top, and 2 servings of 1/4 organic chicken (leg/thigh) with the skin on.
Option 2	An 8-ounce grass-fed steak, 2 cups of sautéed arugula, and 1 cup of steamed brussels sprouts with a sprinkle of sea salt and 1 tablespoon of grass-fed butter on top.

See Chapter 11 for recipes.

IMPROVE YOUR LIVER HEALTH

After taking thousands of students through this protocol, the most common challenge I see is poor liver health, which can be caused from medications, toxins, processed foods, and/or alcohol. The liver produces something called bile acids that help to break down fat-soluble vitamins (A, D, E, and K). When you increase your healthy fats but fail to break them down properly, it causes digestive issues, which lead to loose stools and diarrhea. This can be discouraging and uncomfortable, making it hard to succeed at your reset. The solution? Bitters.

Bitter foods contain antioxidants that can reduce inflammation, improve blood sugar control and insulin sensitivity, boost metabolism in fat cells, and reduce blood pressure. They also support your gut microbiome and may even help protect against cancer.[5]

To make bitter foods more palatable, you can reduce the bitter flavor by leveraging fat to make delicious recipes full of antioxidant-rich vegetables. Bitter foods all contain fat-soluble vitamins (A, D, E, and K) as well as liver-boosting nutrients. Additionally, bitters may increase the production of digestive enzymes, which further aids food absorption. (For more information on supporting your liver, see my book *Metabolic Freedom*.)

Bitter-rich foods to add:

- Arugula
- Organic coffee
- Apple cider vinegar
- Lemons/limes
- Radicchio
- Rosemary
- Thyme
- Basil
- Dill
- Ginger and ginger tea
- Milk thistle tea
- Brussels sprouts
- Broccoli

▲▼▲

Your next step is to build up your metabolic machinery by practicing intermittent-fasting strategies and decreasing dietary fat to prioritize protein. This phase is Pillar 2 (Days 8–21). Let's get started with building your fasting muscle!

CHAPTER SIX

KETO AND FASTING: THE AVOCADO AND EGGS OF WEIGHT LOSS

Before you panic about fasting, think about this: After you've successfully mastered Pillar 1, you've already been fasting for 12 hours a day. I didn't want to call it "fasting," but if you don't eat between dinner at 7 P.M. and breakfast at 7 A.M., you've been fasting. That's why the first meal of the day is called "breakfast." You are literally breaking from your overnight fast. By the way, you don't need to "break your fast" in the morning by loading up on food. This is a Western tradition that's fairly recent in our history. In the medieval era and before, the morning meal was minimal, and what we call "lunch" was the first substantial meal of the day. In fact, eating early in the day was thought to be a sin associated with overindulgence and gluttony. In many cultures—even today—you have only coffee and do not break your fast until noon.

By periodically fasting, you're realigning your digestive system and metabolism to the way we successfully operated for hundreds of thousands of years during the Paleolithic era, when *Homo sapiens* (that's us) were hunter-gatherers. The idea of deliberately planting and harvesting food—what we call the agrarian era—did not enter our brains until the Neolithic Revolution, which started around 10,000 BCE in the Fertile Crescent, the boomerang-shaped region of the Middle East where people first took up farming. Considering that *Homo sapiens* emerged in Africa about 250,000 years ago, that's quite recent!

In this chapter we'll move on to Pillar 2, where we'll begin a longer, more structured window of intermittent fasting. You'll be dialing back your fat intake and focusing instead on hitting your protein requirements. I'll provide you with some tips for successful fasting as well as an advanced reset for those interested.

FASTING INCREASES HUMAN GROWTH HORMONE

The power of fasting lies not in the mere reduction of calories, but in the beneficial hormonal changes. One of the main benefits comes from reducing insulin, but there are also increases in noradrenalin, cortisol, and growth hormone. Collectively, these are known as the counter-regulatory hormones, since they all serve to increase blood glucose at a time when the body is not obtaining glucose from food. Your body's pituitary gland naturally produces human growth hormone (HGH), or somatotropin, which is a peptide hormone that stimulates growth, cell reproduction, and cell regeneration in humans and other animals. It helps to regulate body composition, body fluids, muscle and bone growth, sugar and fat metabolism, and possibly heart function. Beginning in middle age, the pituitary gland slowly reduces the amount of growth hormone it produces.

HGH is also said to benefit the quality and appearance of the skin. This hormone can help to speed up healing after an injury and repair muscle tissue after exercise. It helps to build muscle mass, boost metabolism, and burn fat. It's said to slow down the aging process and treat age-related diseases. Research supporting these claims is ongoing. We do know, however, that fasting is a great stimulus to HGH secretion. During fasting, there is the spike in the early morning, followed by regular secretion throughout the day.

Researchers led by M. L. Hartman also showed a fivefold increase in HGH in response to a two-day fast.[1] They examined how short-term fasting affects endogenous growth hormone (GH) secretion in healthy men. In this landmark human metabolic study, nine normal male subjects were monitored over 24-hour intervals under two conditions: a fed (control) day and then the second day of a 48-hour fast.

The authors measured GH concentrations in blood drawn every five minutes and applied rigorous deconvolution methods to estimate GH secretory bursts, frequency, amplitude, and clearance. The results were remarkable: After just two days without food, participants' natural growth hormone levels increased about fivefold. This surge happened because their bodies started releasing growth hormone more often and in larger amounts each time. In other words, fasting didn't change how fast the body cleared the hormone—it simply made the body produce a lot more of it. This powerful hormonal response helps explain why short fasts can boost fat burning and protect muscle even when you're not eating.

YOUR FASTING SCHEDULE FOR DAYS 8–21

It's time to implement intermittent fasting into your schedule. You can also look at it from the point of view of when you can eat. Another name for this is time-restricted eating (TRE), and it means that you eat only within a window of a certain number of hours a day.

You will be practicing an 18/6 intermittent-fasting schedule during this part of your reset. This means that during 24 hours, you will be in a fasted state for 18 hours and a fed state for 6 hours. For example, your first meal of the day, "break-fast," could be at 12 P.M., and you would finish eating at 6 P.M. Then you would fast from 6 P.M. to 12 P.M. the next day. The actual times you choose to break your fast and finish eating are flexible, as long as you follow the protocol of fasting for 18 hours and eating within that 6-hour window.

During your eating window, you will hit your protein requirement goal and keep your total carbohydrates at the upper limit you found to keep you in ketosis. How do you determine your required protein amount? The first step is to determine your desired goal weight—this is the total body weight you want to achieve. Then you want to consume 1 gram of protein per pound of ideal body weight. For example, if you currently weigh 165 pounds but your ideal body weight is 125 pounds, your protein requirement would be 125 grams per day. You will simultaneously lower your fat intake.

"But Ben, I thought keto was high fat," many people say. It should be in the beginning, but once you're fat adapted, which you should be by now, it's time to let your body tap into body fat for its fat requirements. You can obtain your fat calories from your keto foods—or from your love handles. You're no longer following the 2/2/2/2 rule at this point. There's no need to track fat consumption, so you can stop adding butter and coconut oil to your coffee. There's no total number or percent of fat to hit at this point; simply get the fat that occurs naturally with your protein sources. As far as carbohydrates, you will continue to keep these within your carbohydrate threshold. For some, that's 50 grams or less of carbohydrates per day, while for others it may be 25 grams or less. Testing your blood ketones will help you find this threshold.

THREE HELPFUL TIPS FOR FASTING

Unfortunately, many people who practice fasting do not experience the wonderful benefits it has to offer, because they give up. Why do they give up? They simply don't know the rules. There are three things you can do to make intermittent fasting easier so you can accelerate fat loss and increase mental clarity.

1. **Get fat adapted.** The first way to make intermittent fasting easier for you is to build up your "fasting muscle" by getting fat adapted. You've already achieved this by completing the first seven days in your reset. Good job!

2. **Use fasting crutches!** The second way to obtain better results with fasting is to use fasting crutches if you need to. There are certain beverages and food items you can have during a fast and still maximize its benefits. My favorite fasting crutches are tea, coffee, electrolytes, bone broth (breaks a fast), and fat bombs. Fat bombs are small, high-fat, low-carb snacks—typically made with ingredients like coconut oil, nut butter, and cocoa—that provide quick energy and help keep you in ketosis between meals.

3. **Rethink your "break-fast."** The third way to make fasting easier is to break the fast with mostly protein and fat, not carbohydrates. As you're exiting a fast, be mindful of your blood sugar, and avoid sharp

blood sugar spikes. Immediately following a fast, your body can be highly sensitive to carbohydrates, and added sugars or processed carbohydrates could send your insulin spiking through the roof. Foods to break your fast that support your Keto Flex lifestyle include:

- Beef sticks
- Beef jerky
- Eggs
- Protein shakes
- Sliced deli meats (nitrite-free)
- Chicken breast
- Turkey
- Grass-fed beef
- Bone broth
- High-protein vegetables such as peas, broccoli, mushrooms, and brussels sprouts
- Avocado

FAT ADAPTATION VS. KETO ADAPTATION

Let's quickly clear up a common point of confusion between the terms *fat adapted* and *keto adapted*. *Fat adapted* means your body can convert fat to energy. When you're fat adapted, you don't need a steady stream of glucose to stay active. Instead, during food deprivation your body can access a ready supply of energy in the form of body fat. Then, after the crisis, you can quickly go back to burning carbs.

When you're fat adapted, you can process a load of carbs and then return to burning fat once blood sugar and insulin levels subside. When the metabolism has the flexibility to shift from burning through its sugar reserves to tapping into fat stores, this accelerates fat loss and the benefits of fasting.

Keto adapted is slightly different. It means that being in ketosis—burning fat instead of carbs—is the rule rather than the exception. Fat adaptation can occur to different degrees and across a spectrum dependent on the degree of carb restriction; keto adaptation represents a more comprehensive reshaping of many physiologic systems. Keto adaptation happens only when carbs are restricted to a point that induces sustained nutritional ketosis. Think of being fat adapted as the first (and very positive) step toward better health and loss of excess weight, and being keto adapted as the next step. The goal is to help you achieve keto adaptation by the end of our 45-Day Keto Flex Reset.

ADVANCED KETO RESET FOR PILLAR 2

If you want to obtain even better results from this phase, I encourage you to practice early time-restricted feeding. Studies show that our circadian rhythm and hormones are designed to eat most of our calories during the day. Dr. Courtney Pederson from the University of Birmingham, Alabama, had a fascinating study on early time-restricted feeding.[2] The study had two groups. Both groups consumed the same food and calories, controlled inside a laboratory setting. The only difference between these two groups was that group A consumed all their calories between 8 A.M. and 2 P.M., and group B consumed all their calories between 2 P.M. and 8 P.M.

The researchers measured the sirtuin 1 gene, which protects your DNA against damage and has been called a longevity gene, and they also measured autophagy via the LC3a protein. After just four days, group A, who had an earlier eating window, had 22 percent more autophagy and 11 percent more activation of the SIRT1 gene!

If you feel up to it, during Pillar 2 (Days 8–21), shift your eating window to between 8 A.M. and 2 P.M., and you'll experience better results. If this doesn't work for your schedule, don't worry about it. You'll still benefit from the previous schedule outlined for you.

CHAPTER SEVEN

TOXIN TERMINATOR: IMPLEMENTING THE CARNIVORE DIET TO REMOVE PLANT POISONS

In the Keto Flex Reset, the first pillar called for you to adjust your food choices. You've cut down on your carbs, enabling your body to switch more readily to burning fat for fuel. This process produces ketones, which your cells are happy to use for energy. To amplify the positive effects of the Keto Flex lifestyle, Pillar 2 showed you how to intermittently fast while prioritizing protein. By ensuring that no food energy is being introduced for at least 18 hours every day, you're giving your digestive system time to reset, your insulin levels a chance to subside, and your body more ketones to produce. And remember, all of this is without calorie counting or weighing. You just eat normal keto-friendly meals, focused on protein, within your six-hour, time-restricted window of eating. Now you're ready to enter Pillar 3 of your 45-Day Keto Flex Reset—removing the foods that irritate your gut—to unleash the full power of what this lifestyle can offer you.

In this chapter I'll introduce you to the carnivore diet. "The what?" you say. "Carnivore?" Yes! The word *carnivore* comes from the Latin *carn*, for "flesh." We're talking about meat. Any product that comes directly from a creature that walks, swims, or flies. For some people, the idea of eating nothing but animal products is like a dream come true. For others, it may seem gross. Either way, there's a good reason for it. Now that you've lowered carbohydrates to encourage your body to use fat as fuel, and you're comfortable with that, the next step is to *force* your body to become keto adapted while healing your digestive system. This will take your fat-burning power to the next level!

Protein—or more precisely, the amino acids your body needs to make its own protein molecules—comes from two sources: animals and plants. Not all proteins are created equal. Although animal products contain all nine essential amino acids, nuts (including almonds and cashews) and seeds (like sunflower and pumpkin seeds) do not. As a result, they can't be categorized as complete protein examples. Your body needs essential amino acids in complete protein sources to grow and repair tissue. This is why your protein should come from animal products.

The concept is simple: In Pillar 3 (Phase), you'll eat only animal products.

By providing your body with zero carbs, and hence zero glucose, while still providing more than enough nutrition to keep you mentally and physically active, your liver will have no choice but to crank out the ketones to keep your cells happy. If you eliminate carbs, what are you left with? Fat and protein. That describes a nice, juicy rib eye steak! Periodically cutting all vegetables from your diet also gives your body a chance to detox from "antinutrients," transforming your gut from gassy to glorious.

WHAT ARE ANTINUTRIENTS?

Antinutrients are chemicals found in plants that prevent your body from absorbing essential nutrients from food and being the efficient micronutrient sponge that it was meant to be. People and animals pull the nourishment we need from our surroundings, but as evolution would have it, many plants developed the capacity to fight back. Nutrient-sapping phytochemicals protect tasty edibles from being devoured to the point of extinction. This state-of-the-art defense system taught animals that overconsumption resulted in sickness and sometimes death. Animals either evolved to digest the antinutrient-rich plants, or they stopped eating them.

Eating a steady source of antinutrients can lead to gut issues, inflammation, arthritis, brain fog, and autoimmune conditions. Some people are more sensitive to antinutrients than others. It really comes down to the health of your gut. I have many friends and colleagues who believe a carnivore diet is the only way you should eat, and that this should be a lifelong approach. I don't agree with them. I believe a carnivore diet is a fantastic short-term approach because it removes vegetables that have been poisoning us as we work on building up digestive function.

There are several compounds in the foods we eat classified as antinutrients. Antinutrients are found in their highest concentrations in grains, beans, legumes, and nuts, but they can also be found in leaves, roots, and fruits of certain varieties of plants.

Glucosinolates

Found in cruciferous vegetables (broccoli, brussels sprouts, cabbage), these can prevent the absorption of iodine, which may then interfere with thyroid function and cause goiter. Those already with an iodine deficiency or a condition called hypothyroidism are most susceptible.

Lectins

These are proteins in legumes (beans, peanuts, soybeans), grains, and nightshades that can block the absorption of calcium, iron, phosphorus, and zinc. They stick to your intestinal wall and create intestinal permeability. When food moves through your gastrointestinal tract, it rubs against your gut's lining, causing microtrauma. Usually, your cells repair those bumps and bruises before they become a problem, but lectins interfere with that process. They adhere to the walls of your gut, preventing repair. The ensuing damage causes low-level inflammation in your GI tract.

When you eat a lot of lectins, your gut wall can develop holes, and its contents can then seep into your bloodstream, causing leaky-gut syndrome. Thousands of varieties of lectins exist in most plant species. Not all of them are toxic or cause intestinal damage. Some plants contain drastically more lectins than other food sources do, which is why wheat, beans, quinoa, peas, peanuts, white potatoes, tomatoes, and eggplants are suspect. The more you eat, the more damage you may be causing to your body. Instead, concentrate on getting most of your nutrients from foods that come with low risk.

Lectin sensitivity varies widely person to person. You may be able to eat lectins morning, noon, and night, and never have a problem, while your friend can't touch them. You'll know you have a problem with lectins if you experience inflammation, brain fog, migraines, stomach issues, acne, or joint pain after eating a lectin-rich meal. The lectins in nightshades, in particular, are a common autoimmune trigger and can cause sensitivities in many people. To test yourself, fill up on a nightshade-heavy lunch—we're talking about tomatoes, peppers, and potatoes—and see how you feel afterward.

Oxalates

Found in green, leafy vegetables and tea, oxalates (also referred to as oxalic acid) can bind to calcium and prevent it from being absorbed. They can be found in plant sources such as fruits, vegetables, nuts, and seeds. Oxalates can also be produced naturally by your own body.

They often bind to minerals such as calcium and are excreted out of the body through the stool. However, high amounts of oxalate can build up in the kidneys, leading to the formation of kidney stones, which occur when hard mineral deposits form within the inner lining of the kidneys, causing symptoms like stomach pain, nausea, and vomiting.

Phytates (Phytic Acid)

Phytates in whole grains, seeds, legumes, and some nuts can decrease the absorption of iron, zinc, magnesium, and calcium. Phytic acid binds to these minerals, preventing their absorption, so you get little nutrition from the food.

Phytates also inhibit the digestive enzymes pepsin, trypsin, and amylase. Trypsin and pepsin are involved in the breakdown of protein, while amylase is required for the breakdown of starch. When those enzymes aren't present in the right amounts, food doesn't get processed properly, and your body misses out on key nutrients. Think about it like this: If your body has an overload of phytates, while there are fewer nutrients to go around, the body is also substantially less efficient at breaking down macronutrients into their components.

Your body can handle some amount of phytates, but it's a good idea to eliminate the main sources so your minerals will be absorbed. Besides, removing them from your diet completely would be impossible. To build muscle or burn fat, your body needs a certain amount of protein or carbohydrates. It largely depends on how healthy your gut is, because an optimized digestive system requires less food to fuel the body properly.

Gluten

This is the generic name for proteins found in wheat, rye, barley, and oats. In the digestion of most proteins, the long strands are broken down by digestive enzymes, which cleave or break off groups of amino acids called peptides. The majority of these peptides can be further broken down, absorbed through the intestine, and then transported and used in the body. Gluten is an exception—it cannot be broken down by the digestive enzymes. As a result, it can cause intestinal permeability (aka leaky gut).

In terms of how people react to the indigestibility of gluten, they fall into two categories: celiac or nonceliac gluten sensitivity. Most of the gluten-sensitive population belong to the latter group, which means they do not test positive for celiac disease but nonetheless suffer an adverse immune response to gluten, which takes the form of inflammation. Inflammation is generally the culprit behind our gluten-induced brain fog, digestive discomfort, and suboptimal nutrient absorption.

Gluten is hidden in places beyond the obvious sources of bread and pasta. Products like soy sauce, beer, and even processed meats contain gluten that may be downgrading your performance.

Saponins

Also selectively referred to as triterpene glycosides, saponins are bitter-tasting, usually toxic, plant-derived organic chemicals that have a foamy quality when agitated in water. In fact, they are produced by plants as a method of natural pest control. Their bitter taste makes the plant less palatable to birds, insects, and humans.

Saponins are naturally present in quinoa and many other foods, including a wide variety of legumes; vegetables such as spinach, asparagus, beets, garlic, onions, and yams; as well as herbs like ginseng, licorice root, fenugreek, and alfalfa. Many people believe saponins irritate the intestinal lining, causing inflammation and all kinds of other trouble. However, other clinical studies have suggested that saponins can affect the immune system in ways that help to protect the human body against cancers and also reduce cholesterol levels, decrease blood lipids, and lower blood glucose response.[1]

Tannins (or Tannoids)

A class of astringent, polyphenolic biomolecules, tannins bind to and precipitate proteins and various other organic compounds, including amino acids and alkaloids. Like saponins, plants contain tannins to make themselves unpalatable and to deter animals from eating a plant's fruit or seeds before they are ripe. Tannins are responsible for that astringent, mouth-coating feeling you get from biting into an unripe pear or plum. Tannins in tea, coffee, and legumes can decrease iron absorption.

DOES EATING RED MEAT CAUSE CANCER?

You will most likely find yourself eating more red meat during this pillar. Many people believe that eating red meat causes cancer. This is what the mainstream news would like for you to believe. There are numerous studies disproving this myth. Despite what mainstream headlines suggest, the science linking red meat to cancer is far from settled. The studies that often make these claims are largely observational or epidemiological—meaning they can show only associations, not cause and effect. Many of these analyses rely on food-frequency questionnaires, which are notoriously inaccurate and subject to recall bias. People who eat more meat in these studies also tend to engage in other lifestyle factors—like smoking, drinking, eating processed carbs, or avoiding exercise—that confound the results. Even large meta-analyses that suggest a connection often include processed meats and refined-food patterns, not clean, grass-fed red meat. When we look beyond these population-based correlations to controlled trials and clinical data, the picture changes entirely. In my experience working with thousands of people through my programs, I've seen the opposite: When individuals include high-quality, nose-to-tail animal foods, their inflammation markers drop, insulin sensitivity improves, and metabolic health thrives. Real food from healthy animals doesn't promote disease—it helps prevent it.

AUTOIMMUNE BENEFITS FROM THE CARNIVORE DIET

I have Raynaud's autoimmune syndrome, which causes decreased blood flow to the fingers. In some people, it also causes less blood flow to the ears, toes, nipples, knees, or nose. This occurs due to spasms of blood vessels in those areas. The exact cause of Raynaud's is unknown. It's possible that some blood disorders may cause Raynaud's by increasing the blood thickness. This may happen due to excess platelets or red blood cells. Or special receptors in the blood that control the narrowing of the blood vessels may be more sensitive. If you want to know more about Raynaud's syndrome, just Google it, and look at some of the photos. It can be rather mild or really gross and nasty!

As for me, I often experienced a flare-up after eating a meal, and my fingers would become swollen, red, and inflamed. During my 40-day carnivore diet, I had only two small flare-ups. It seemed amazing! As emerging evidence suggests, the carnivore diet has profound benefits on healing the gut.

Raynaud's syndrome is just one of many modern syndromes that seem to plague industrialized nations. From chronic fatigue syndrome to irritable bowel syndrome, we seem to have a global problem with autoimmune disorders. According to the National Institutes of Health, over 23 million people in the United States alone are diagnosed with autoimmune disease, while millions more suffer undiagnosed. In response, doctors prescribe medicine cabinets full of pharmaceuticals, each one aimed at suppressing a particular group of symptoms. This approach often makes things worse as a host of side effects mingle with the already debilitating symptoms.

While clinical research on the subject needs to be conducted, there's growing anecdotal evidence that the carnivore diet has a positive effect on autoimmune diseases, including Raynaud's syndrome. In fact, "meat heals" has become a popular tagline within the carnivore diet community. There is a theory that some people—perhaps myself included—have an extreme or allergic reaction to common plant toxins, including saponins and tannins, which we've discussed in this chapter.

If you suffer from a stubborn autoimmune disease that defies a cure, why not follow the carnivore diet for a few weeks? You may discover surprising results.

YOUR EATING AND FASTING PATTERN FOR DAYS 22–45

Survival is the number-one priority for the primal brain, and it will do anything to support that. Major dietary shifts drive survival adaptation mechanisms. To survive changes, the body drives hormonal optimization, making hormones more sensitive and increasing growth hormone. As we learned in Chapter 6, growth hormone is an anti-aging, healing, and fat-burning hormone. During this process the body changes its genetic expression and strengthens the microbiome.

Here's the rule: During periods of adaptation, good cells get stronger, while bad cells don't adapt. We want our cells to become stronger, not sicker.

In our modern industrialized society, where we have all the food we could possibly want, how do we make our primal brain happy? *Diet variation* is where the magic happens. I discovered this concept from my health mentor, Dr. Daniel Pompa. We can mimic the conditions of our ancient existence by forcing changes in our diet. Adapt or die, baby! It's a wonderful process. Diet variation is so magical because when you change your diet, your body is forced to adapt. There's not one ancient culture in the history of the world that stuck with one diet their entire life cycle; it just didn't happen.

Remember, the foundation of the Keto Flex lifestyle is to starve your body of carbs that can be turned into glucose. In the absence of glucose, we want the body to activate the ready supply of stored energy in your fat cells. In this way, you'll shed the excess fat and be leaner and healthier. The best way to ease into the Keto Flex lifestyle is to follow the traditional approach of boosting your fat intake while lowering your consumption of protein and carbs. Once you're accustomed to that approach, to keep your primal brain happy and to take that next step to *zero* carbs, you need to switch it up and shift to a protein-heavy diet. This will keep you feeling full, trick your primal brain into thinking you're adapting to changing conditions, and shut off the supply of carbs, forcing your body to switch to ketones for energy. Pretty neat, isn't it? You don't do a carnivore diet forever, because the key to success is constant change and metabolic flexibility.

During Days 22–45 of Pillar 3, you'll choose between four different levels of the carnivore diet:

Level 1:

- Grass-fed-and-finished beef, beef tallow, and salt

Level 2:

- Grass-fed-and-finished beef, beef tallow, and salt
- Grass-fed-and-finished lamb
- Wild-caught seafood
- Grass-fed-and-finished bison
- Organic, pastured pork and bacon
- Organic, free-range poultry
- Free-range rabbit, elk, and venison
- Organ meat

Level 3:

- Grass-fed-and-finished beef, beef tallow, and salt
- Grass-fed-and-finished lamb
- Wild-caught seafood
- Grass-fed-and-finished bison
- Organic, pastured pork and bacon
- Organic, free-range poultry
- Free-range rabbit, elk, and venison
- Organ meat
- Grass-fed dairy (sheep and goat are preferred)
- Pastured-raised, free-range eggs

Level 4:

- Grass-fed-and-finished beef, beef tallow, and salt
- Grass-fed-and-finished lamb
- Wild-caught seafood
- Grass-fed-and-finished bison
- Organic, pastured pork and bacon
- Organic, free-range poultry
- Free-range rabbit, elk, and venison
- Organ meat
- Grass-fed dairy (sheep and goat are preferred)
- Pastured-raised, free-range eggs
- Raw honey
- Spices
- Low-sugar, plant-based sauces (Primal Kitchen, Chosen Foods, etc.)

Which level should you follow? For my clients who have severe autoimmune disease, I put them on Level 1. This is the most restrictive, but it achieves serious results. If you don't have a severe autoimmune disease, you can choose whichever level feels comfortable. I've had students do Level 4 for a week, Level 3 for a week, and so on.

It's important to note that the quality of the animals you eat should be considered. I personally have my animal products shipped to me from Wild Pastures. These are clean animal products from animals on regenerative farms. If you head to http://www.benazadi.com/meat, you can get 20 percent off your first box plus a $15 bonus.

You're also going to mix things up with your intermittent-fasting schedule to keep the body guessing and adapting. Here's your new fasting schedule for Pillar 3.

Days 22–28: For the first seven days of Pillar 3, follow a 20/4 schedule: 20 hours fasting, 4 hours carnivore feasting. This could look like: At 12 P.M. you break your fast. By 4 P.M. you're done eating for the day. This means you're fasting between 4 P.M. one day and 12 P.M. the next day, having only water and sea salt. You'll be eating carnivore during your 4-hour eating window; choose any level you'd like.

Days 29–45: After you complete the 20/4 fasting schedule for seven days, follow an alternate-day fasting schedule. You're going to combine alternate-day fasting with OMAD (one meal a day). Here's what this part of Pillar 3 looks like on your calendar:

Day 29: Eat three carnivore meals: breakfast, lunch, and dinner (no fasting)

Day 30: Complete a 24-hour fast, consuming one carnivore meal (OMAD)

Day 31: Eat 3 carnivore meals: breakfast, lunch, and dinner (no fasting)

Day 32: Complete a 24-hour fast, consuming one carnivore meal (OMAD)

You'll continue with this alternate-day fasting schedule until Day 45.

Once you complete this, you move to Pillar 4: Flex. You can also choose to continue this carnivore pillar for a few more weeks. Your race, your pace!

One Meal a Day (OMAD)

The more you learn about the keto lifestyle, the more you'll see the acronym *OMAD*. It stands for "one meal a day." One of the interesting aspects of the Keto Flex lifestyle is that instead of feeling like you're starving, which is a feature of most other diets, you're more likely to feel physiologically satiated. When the opportunity to eat presents itself on your schedule, instead of feeling like a happy pig headed for the slop trough to gorge, you're more likely to feel like a finicky house cat who acts like food is a necessary annoyance. (If you've ever owned a cat, you know what I mean!) You won't be going crazy for food.

In my own experience on the Keto Flex lifestyle, I generally feel physiologically satisfied—even on one meal a day—but sometimes psychologically unsatisfied. This is simply because eating is a pleasurable experience, and going 23 hours with nothing but water and salt is, well, a little boring at first. But after a while, you get used to it, and it feels more like freedom. You don't have to worry about eating . . . or even think about it. You just keep going, like the Energizer Bunny.

The OMAD approach may remind you of the "warrior diet." Popularized in the book *The Warrior Diet* by Ori Hofmekler, the diet is based on the idea that ancient warriors had no time to eat because they were too busy rampaging and pillaging, so they ate one big meal before bedtime and then nothing but incidental snacks and water for the following 23 hours. The book shamelessly flatters its readers by proclaiming they can be "predator/victors," and that Hofmekler himself is a magnificent human specimen. I'm sure that's true, but the problem many people have is that the warrior diet encourages you to eat as much food as you can of any type during that one meal and then sleep it off overnight like a lion sleeps after making a big kill. To improve your body composition and overall health for the better, you need to be mindful of the quality of your diet.

More scientific research is needed on the effects of OMAD. The only study that I know on OMAD was published in 2007. Entitled "A Controlled Trial of Reduced Meal Frequency Without Caloric Restriction in Healthy, Normal-Weight, Middle-Aged Adults," for two eight-week periods, the researchers allowed the test group to take the "warrior" approach and eat the equivalent of three meals in just one meal per day, meaning their total calorie intake over 24 hours was the same as that of the three-meal-a-day control group. Not unexpectedly, no weight loss was reported.[2]

Alternate-Day Fasting

In alternate-day fasting, you fast every other day. A full fast every other day can seem extreme, so it's not recommended for beginners. You may go to bed very hungry several times per week, which is challenging and probably unsustainable in the long term. Therefore, some versions allow about 500 calories during the fasting days.

Eat-Fast-Eat

This diet, popularized by fitness expert Brad Pilon, involves a 24-hour fast two or three times per week. Basically, you eat one day, fast the next day, and eat on the third day. Then you repeat the pattern—eat, fast, eat. Water, coffee, and other zero-calorie beverages are allowed during the fast, but no solid foods are permitted.[3]

Because each week has an odd number of days, the eating/fasting days of the week will rotate. If you fast on Tuesday and Friday of the first week, then in the second week, you'll fast on Monday, Thursday, and Sunday.

By fasting from dinner one day to dinner the next day, this amounts to a full 24-hour fast. You can also fast from breakfast to breakfast or lunch to lunch—the end result is the same. But you need to be consistent and fast for a full 24 hours each time.

An important note: You will not be hitting your protein requirements on your OMAD days, and that's okay short term, as your body will get rid of *junky* protein. If you're having a hard time hitting your protein requirements on non-OMAD days, then aim to get at least 40 grams of protein at each meal.

IF YOU'RE NOT FEELING WELL ON CARNIVORE

- You may be eating meat that is very lean. Switch to fattier cuts of meat. This can also be beneficial if you're dealing with constipation.
- Add 1 to 3 teaspoons of raw honey around exercise time and/or before sleep.
- Keep your electrolytes and minerals up.
- Be patient. Your body will adapt!

▲▼▲

As I mentioned, if you need more time on Pillar 3, that's fine! We don't want to arouse the ire of your primal-brain watchdog. Just keep at it. You'll find that the fewer carbs and sugars you eat, the less you'll want them. If you'd like support from me, and a community of like-minded individuals, I encourage you to become a member of the Fat Loss Academy. As a member, you'll have access to on-demand videos structured in a step-by-step system to master these four pillars. This is a great way to keep yourself accountable on your Keto Flex lifestyle. Visit fatlossacademy.com to become a member today.

CHAPTER EIGHT

MASTERING THE ART OF KETO FLEXIBILITY

Consuming a low number of carbohydrates over the long term is a good thing, because you'll burn excess body fat and improve your overall health. But there's one important caveat: A constant, unrelenting state of ketosis—in which your body is burning its own fat for fuel—is unsustainable, because eventually you'd have no more fat. We've now moved into Pillar 4, where you'll flex in and out of keto, enjoy feast days, and master your body's ability to adapt. The Flex pillar will allow you to maintain your keto lifestyle month after month, year after year.

In this chapter I'll outline seven reasons why long-term ketosis is bad for your body to better illustrate why flexing in and out of keto is your best tool for long-term health. I'll explain the right ways to incorporate your feast days and provide some simple eating/fasting schedules you can follow. Finally, I'll teach you how to adapt the program if you are diabetic. One caveat: If you're a woman, don't follow the eating/fasting schedules at the end of this chapter. Instead, when you get to that section, skip ahead to Chapter 9, where I have a special flex plan just for you.

SEVEN REASONS WHY LONG-TERM KETOSIS IS A BAD IDEA

My mantra is "Lose the excess fat; treasure the necessary fat." Ketosis is a brilliant strategy for accomplishing the first goal. As for the second goal, prolonged ketosis doesn't have an automatic shut-off valve. If you remain in a state of constant ketosis, your body will continue burning your own fat as long as it must to stay alive. When you have no more fat left to burn, various bodily functions will be shut off or minimized. This process of shutting down will continue until Mr. Death knocks on your door and says, "Sorry, buddy—time's up." No one wants that.

Your ultimate goal is to achieve metabolic flexibility. In the United States, 93 percent of adults are metabolically inflexible; in other words, their metabolism is stuck burning sugar/glucose in a keto deficiency. On the flip side, we have the people in the keto space who have done keto for too long, and they have created another form of metabolic inflexibility where their metabolism is stuck burning fat/ketones and forgotten about sugar/glucose. A healthy metabolism has the ability to move back and forth between burning sugar and burning fat, without a hiccup. Keto flexing is how to achieve this process of long-term metabolic flexibility. It's important to detach the dogma from keto and view it as a metabolic tool in your health shed, but not the *only* tool!

Most of our real data is what we've seen clinically. I work alongside 47-plus doctors, including Dr. Daniel Pompa and many others. Combined, we have a patient and client population of more than 100,000 people. Every week, we do case studies with patients/clients. Some of our observations include:

- Keto works well for teaching the cells to choose a cleaner source (really important for detox).
- Men can be more aggressive with keto than women.
- Cycling women need to be more strategic, and flex in and out more often (more on this in Chapter 9).
- People who do strict keto long term (six months straight or longer) experience issues with their thyroid, sex hormone binding globulin (SHBG), free testosterone, cortisol, and glucose numbers.

We are huge fans of the DUTCH hormone test, and we use the blood markers we spoke about earlier in the book, the Oura ring to measure heart rate variability, and continuous glucose monitors. If someone is doing keto long term, and all their markers look great and they feel fantastic, then they should probably continue.

To ensure that you're well informed, let's review some of the bad things that can happen if you go too far with ketosis.

1. The Metabolism Panics and Fat Burning Slows Down

As levels of body fat drop, your primal brain—whom we thought we had trained to accept a high-fat diet and fasting—will be aroused and begin to object. That eternal watchdog will sense that your reserves of fat are becoming depleted. Remembering those long periods of deprivation thousands of years ago, it will sound the alarm: *The fat supply is running low!* It will issue the command that your body must preserve its precious fuel. In response, your body will actually slow down fat burning—all for the sake of survival!

When you stay in ketosis too long, the body starts to rebel and conserve its fuel. Imagine if you lived out in the woods and had stored 500 logs of firewood to heat your cabin for the winter. These were your reserves, because you could still go out and chop more firewood. So, if you had to dip into these reserves, you wouldn't be worried. But now it's early March, and snow still covers the ground. It's been a tough winter, you haven't harvested many trees, and you see that you have only 50 logs left. That's a low supply! Suddenly you're reluctant to use them, because you don't want to run out. When you had 500 logs, you didn't care about burning them.

The same thing happens with your body fat. This is why when you remain on a low-carbohydrate diet for too long, your body will *slow down* fat metabolism.

And you know what? This is a good thing. There's a big difference between losing *excess* fat and losing *all* your fat. You want to lose excess fat. But your body needs a small amount of fat, and your primal brain is smart to insist that you meet this minimal requirement.

2. Thyroid Problems

Hormone production is often a "chain of command," as orders are passed from one organ to another, until the desired outcome is achieved. The hypothalamus and the pituitary gland, which are located in the brain, help control the thyroid, a butterfly-shaped gland located at the base of your throat, just below the Adam's apple. To provide their direction to the thyroid, the hypothalamus releases thyrotropin-releasing hormone (TRH), which stimulates the pituitary gland to release thyroid-stimulating hormone (TSH). When the hypothalamus and pituitary are working normally, they respond when thyroid hormone levels are low, secreting more TRH and TSH, which stimulates the thyroid to make more hormones. When thyroid hormone levels are too high, they secrete less TRH and TSH, which reduces hormone production by the thyroid.

The thyroid gland uses iodine from food to make two thyroid hormones: triiodothyronine (T3) and thyroxine (T4). The primary secretory product is inactive thyroxine (T4), which is a prohormone of triiodothyronine (T3). T4 is converted to T3 peripherally by tissues with high blood flow, including the liver and kidneys. In the brain, T4 is converted to active T3 by type II deiodinase produced by glial cells. The thyroid stores T3 and T4 and releases them when they are needed. These two thyroid hormones function in almost every cell in your body and play a fundamental role in regulating your metabolism and maintaining your resting energy expenditure—that is, the energy you burn just to keep functioning while sitting on the sofa.

Diet can influence thyroid hormone levels, and prolonged ketosis and severe calorie restriction can lead to reduced thyroid function, or hypothyroidism, which is a mechanism to ensure survival in response to perceived famine. The goal is to slow metabolism, conserve energy, and preserve vital organs.

T4 is the inactive form of thyroid; it needs to be converted to T3, which is the active form used by the cells. Do you know which hormone helps with this conversion? Insulin. Low thyroid hormones cause a drop in insulin levels, the hormone needed to transport sugar from the blood to different cells throughout the body. Chronic low insulin levels slow down cellular function, including muscle contractions and basic brain function. Over longer periods of time, low insulin levels compromise this T4 to T3 thyroid hormone conversion.

3. Testosterone Deficiency

Sex hormone binding globulin (SHBG) is a protein made by your liver. It binds tightly to three sex hormones found in both men and women: estrogen, dihydrotestosterone (DHT), and testosterone. SHBG carries these three hormones throughout your blood. It controls the amount of testosterone that your body tissues can use, and too little testosterone in men and too much testosterone in women can cause problems. Factors such as sex, age, obesity, liver disease, and hypothyroidism can change the level of SHBG in your blood. What I've seen reviewing lab work over the years is that too much SHBG leads to lower testosterone levels, and not enough SHBG leads to an increase in estrogen; both can be problematic for men and women. Long-term ketosis can lead to either of these.

4. Leptin Reset

Leptin is your "stop eating!" hormone, and it plays an instrumental role in your hunger and weight management. It comes from the Greek word *leptos,* meaning "thin." Fat cells produce leptin in proportion to levels of body fat: The more fat cells you have, the more leptin they make. When your body fat increases, your leptin levels rise. Your brain senses the increase in leptin and thinks, *Okay, we've got enough fat in reserve, so we can stop eating.* Thus, you eat less and burn more. Conversely, when you don't eat, your body fat decreases, leading your leptin levels to drop. Your brain, sensing a shortage of leptin, thinks, *Hmm, we're low on fat reserves. Better find some food!* At that point, you eat more and burn less. This negative feedback loop is similar to the control mechanisms for many physiological functions, such as body temperature, breathing, and blood pressure.

A properly working leptin system tells your brain that you have enough energy stored in your fat cells to engage in normal, everyday metabolic processes. It leads to better brain function, memory, metabolic performance, mental sharpness, and coordination, and it can even affect the regulation of mood and emotion.

Unfortunately, many overweight people suffer from *leptin resistance*. They have plenty of blood leptin, but the brain doesn't recognize it. Despite the abundance of leptin, the brain thinks there is too little leptin—and orders the body to *keep eating!* This is obviously a bad situation. What causes it? Several potential mechanisms have been identified:

- **Free fatty acids.** Having elevated free fatty acids in your bloodstream may increase fat metabolites in your brain and interfere with leptin signaling.
- **Inflammation.** Inflammatory signaling in your hypothalamus could be a cause of leptin resistance.
- **Consistently high leptin.** It may be that your brain gets accustomed to a constant flood of leptin churned out by your fat cells and becomes "numb" to it.

So, what happens when you follow a low-carb keto diet that puts you in long-term ketosis? Perhaps paradoxically, many people do not suffer from an increase in appetite, as you might expect from falling levels of leptin. It's complicated, but the short version of the story is that leptin levels will drop, which would normally signal your brain to start eating. But something else happens—your brain becomes more sensitive to the effects of leptin, so a smaller amount of leptin packs more punch. In addition, the brain's response to leptin is inhibited by inflammation, resulting in increased leptin resistance. Obesity increases inflammation, which increases the brain's "numbness" to high levels of leptin. Inflammation is dramatically reduced by sustained nutritional ketosis. The reduction in leptin resistance due to reduced inflammation adds to the brain's heightened sensitivity to leptin. In other words, on a well-formulated ketogenic diet the brain perceives a *greater* satiety response to *less* leptin. This explains the paradox as to why we see a decrease in appetite with nutritional ketosis.

To achieve a sustained state of ketosis, you need to occasionally boost your levels of leptin and send the signal to your brain that higher levels of leptin are normal, and that you need to keep eating. This is another reason why the "flex" part of the Keto Flex lifestyle is so important.

We never want your brain to think you're starving—but we also don't want it to forget about eating!

5. Adrenal and Cortisol Issues

We've already made the case that a metabolic state of ketosis is considered a stress to the body through the principle of hormesis. Short term, this is a positive stress that helps you become healthier and stronger. But when you're in a continuous state of ketosis, this stress is too much for your body to adapt to.

The reason for this has to do with cortisol. When you chronically lower glucose and insulin levels through long-term ketosis, your body will release cortisol to stimulate the production of glucose by your liver. Cortisol also promotes inflammation and central obesity, so you don't want chronically elevated cortisol levels.

Your body is going to compensate by self-generating glucose, and that stimulus to make glucose is part of the obesity puzzle, because one of the ways in which your body produces glucose is by secreting cortisol. If your cortisol is chronically elevated, you end up with central obesity and chronic inflammation, which clearly isn't good.

So, if you're not eating enough glucose, your body will make it. And, in fact, the primary evolutionary role of cortisol—the acute role—is actually preventing blood glucose from dropping too low, because that will put you into a hypoglycemic coma. In the longer run its secondary role is to reduce inflammation. So really, the acute, lifesaving role of cortisol on a daily basis is to prevent you from falling into a coma because your blood glucose plunged too low.

When you're increasing the carbohydrate intake, you should be decreasing the amount of fat. If you're not, then at least you should be taking something that stimulates the oxidation of carbohydrates so that it doesn't result in raising triglycerides.

6. Physiological Insulin Resistance

There's a lot of chatter on the Internet about keto causing insulin resistance and type 2 diabetes. How could this be if we just made the case that keto has been proven to reverse insulin resistance and type

2 diabetes? One reason for higher-than-expected fasting glucose is something called *physiological insulin resistance*. This is a phenomenon that occurs in people who've followed keto for a significant length of time. In people who are keto adapted, they've adhered to a very low carbohydrate intake for a long time—most of the body's cells run happily on fatty acids and ketones, with a much lower requirement for glucose than in people on a higher-carb diet. Since these cells are fueled effectively and efficiently by fats and ketones, they need only minimal glucose.

The majority of glucose is spared for tissues with an absolute requirement for it, such as the brain. With muscle tissue "refusing" the glucose to keep it available for the brain, the blood glucose rises, especially first thing in the morning. This is sometimes called physiological insulin resistance to differentiate it from *pathological* insulin resistance, but a better name for it is *adaptive glucose sparing*—an adaptation some people's bodies make. Some keto experts refer to this as a healthy, normal, and to-be-expected response to a very low carbohydrate intake, but there are some who think this can be problematic.

Long-term ketosis tells the mitochondria to protect themselves at all costs and to stop making muscle protein. It also tells them to produce insulin resistance so the muscle doesn't steal any glucose that the brain needs. This is why hard-core keto dieters have higher glucose levels.

7. Possible Cancer

Keto naysayers say "keto causes cancer" because of the slow buildup of the nasty free radical 4-hydroxynonenal (4-HNE) in the body with long-term ketosis. I think they're just hating on keto, but there's some validity to the 4-HNE buildup. This is more likely with people consuming a lot of inflammatory fats on keto (remember those seed oils I told you to avoid?).

Lipid peroxidation generates 4-hydroxynonenal, a key factor in cancer progression. A review by Françoise Guéraud emphasizes 4-HNE's impact on mitochondria, crucial for cellular energy and cancer metabolism.[1] 4-HNE disrupts mitochondrial function, impairing energy production and increasing reactive oxygen species (ROS), contributing to genomic instability and tumor growth. Additionally, it alters mitochondrial dynamics, affecting cellular bioenergetics and promoting a tumor-supportive environment. Understanding 4-HNE's role in mitochondrial dysfunction offers insights for targeted cancer therapies.

These findings suggest that the ketogenic diet could actually serve as an effective addition to cancer treatment by promoting mitochondrial 4-HNE formation, oxidative stress, and lipid peroxidation.

The lipid oxidation product 4-hydroxynonenal has various effects by binding to proteins, impacting multiple cellular pathways associated with cancer. The detoxification of HNE, coordinated by the Nrf2 pathway, plays a crucial role in determining its effects on cells. The bottom line: If you're consuming healthy fats on keto versus the inflammatory ones, and practicing the Keto Flex approach, I don't think you need to worry about keto causing cancer.

THE KETO FLEX SOLUTION: FEAST DAYS

What can you do to reassure your primal brain that you aren't going to starve to death? You give it a little of what it wants—a *feast day!* Hence the term *keto flex*. The "flex" part is very important.

I love keto flexing, because you teach your body to have hormone flexibility, as well as to be able to switch back and forth between burning fat and glucose. Remember, in our industrialized culture, we have to make a conscious effort to follow such a diet plan; for hundreds of thousands of years, our ancestors didn't have to make a conscious effort, because this was normal life. Food was available intermittently, and fasting wasn't "fasting"; it was just those regular periods during which no food was available, or it had to be rationed. They didn't think about it—they just did it. If you killed a deer and you knew that deer had to feed your family for a month, would you eat the whole thing in one week? Of course not. You'd smoke the meat and then dole it out a little bit at a time.

Important Keto Flex (Feast Day) Tip

When you're increasing your carbohydrate intake on a keto flex day, you should be decreasing the amount of fat. Keto flex days are low-fat days. If you decide to eat both energy sources daily (even quality carbohydrates and fats), you activate the Randle cycle. When the Randle cycle is constantly "on," your cells will self-preserve by blocking the efficient use of fatty acids and the use of glucose. This causes fats to pool up in your bloodstream, leading to high levels of an inflammatory molecule called lipopolysaccharide (LPS), which increases insulin resistance, metabolic syndrome, and obesity. The first sign of this happening is an increase in your blood triglycerides.

With the pages ahead, I've made sure to customize your schedule so this doesn't happen. If you've built your metabolic machinery using the first three pillars as your guide, then you should be back in a fat-burning, ketogenic state within 24 hours after a Keto Flex feast day.

Eating/Fasting Schedules

Here are a few eating/fasting schedules that you can follow. See which one works for you or vary them! All that matters is that you shut off the food spigot on a regular basis for an extended period of time—at least 12 hours, but ideally for 16 or 24 hours. You can find a list of healthy carbohydrate flex-day foods in Appendix B.

Weekly 5-1-1

This seven-day method is a good approach if you've achieved your ideal body weight by the end of Pillar 3, or if you want to put on healthy weight.

5 days of intermittent fasting for 16 to 20 hours. When you're eating during the 4-to-8-hour window, stick to keto-friendly meals, with an emphasis on hitting your protein requirement. Eat less than 50 grams of total carbohydrates.

1 24-hour water-only fast day (for example, dinner to dinner).

1 feast (flex) day. Have three meals of high (healthy) carbohydrates and protein. Consume between 100 to 150 grams of healthy carbs and protein. Eat less fat on this day. Aim to keep your total grams of fat under 40.

Weekly 4-2-1

This method is good if you still have 5 to 20 pounds to lose.

4 days of intermittent fasting for 16 to 20 hours. When you're eating during the 4-to-8-hour window, stick to keto-friendly meals. Eat less than 30 grams of total carbohydrates and hit your protein requirement.

2 days of a 48-hour water-only fast.

1 feast (flex) day. Have three meals of high (healthy) carbohydrates and protein. Consume 100 to 150 grams of healthy carbs and protein. Eat less fat on this day. Aim to keep your total grams of fat under 40.

Weekly 3-3-1

This method is good if you still have 20 pounds or more to lose.

3 days of intermittent fasting for 16 to 20 hours. When you're eating during the 4-to-8-hour window, stick to keto-friendly meals. Eat less than 30 grams of total carbohydrates and hit your protein requirement.

3 days of a 72-hour water-only fast.

1 feast (flex) day. Have three meals of high (healthy) carbohydrates and protein. Consume 100 to 150 grams of healthy carbs and protein. Eat less fat on this day. Aim to keep your total grams of fat under 40.

HOW TO KETO FLEX IF YOU'RE DIABETIC

The goal is metabolic flexibility over dogma. If you've completed your 45-Day Keto Flex Reset and you still have type 2 diabetes or prediabetes, you may want to stay in ketosis longer as you work on reversing it. You can repeat the entire 45-Day Keto Flex Reset or continue with Pillar 3 until you've seen significant improvements with your blood values.

If you choose to flex, here's a protocol that can work well. I highly encourage you to work with your health practitioner. As you become healthier, you'll work with your prescribing doctor to lower your meds and eventually eliminate them completely.

4-2-1 Rule for Diabetics

4 days of intermittent fasting for 16 to 20 hours. When you're eating during the 4-to-8-hour window, stick to keto-friendly meals focused on protein. Eat less than 20 grams of total carbohydrates and hit your protein requirement outlined earlier in this book.

2 days of a 48-hour water-only fast.

1 feast (flex) day. Instead of raising your carbohydrates, you will increase your caloric and protein load. Consume 1.2 grams of protein per pound of ideal body weight. For example, if your goal weight is 180 pounds, you will consume 216 grams of protein on this day (180 x 1.2). Bump up your fats to increase your caloric load. Keep total carbohydrates under 30 grams for this day.

Remember, what you eat at meals is extremely important. While you want to consume some carbs to maintain a supply of fat cells and ensure your body can switch back and forth between burning fat and glucose, a diet of crappy, sugary, processed foods will destroy the progress you've made. To stay healthy, eat healthy!

I'm on a mission to reverse type 2 diabetes in 1 billion people in the next 10 years. My client John struggled with high blood pressure, obesity, and type 2 diabetes for six years. After following my advice, he was able to put his diabetes into remission within just 12 weeks. John lost over 130 pounds and came off long-term medication through accountability, consistency, discipline, and patience. His remarkable transformation is proof that it's never too late to reclaim your health. If you have prediabetes or diabetes, or know someone who does, please visit benazadi.com to learn more.

▲▼▲

Now let's talk about customizing a Keto Flex approach for both menstruating and postmenopausal women. The next chapter is the complete guide to keto and fasting for women. If you're a man, don't skip the next chapter. You have relationships with women in your life, and the better you can understand their hormones, the better your relationships will be.

CHAPTER NINE

THE CUSTOMIZED KETO FLEX PLAN FOR WOMEN

What you've learned so far is that there is no cookie-cutter approach to keto and fasting. You're as unique as a snowflake. I want to share a quick story to emphasize this. Every week, a teenage boy would walk by and see an artist going to work chipping away at a piece of stone. Several weeks into this, the artist had carved out a Greek god, a beautiful masterpiece of art. The teenage boy was astonished by what this artist was able to accomplish. The boy walked up to the artist and said, "Mister, how did you know this person was in there?" The artist looked at him, smiled, and said, "Young man, he was in there the entire time." Every human being has unique, individual biochemical needs. Why is the Mona Lisa so expensive? Because the Mona Lisa is one of a kind. And so are you! You are a masterpiece because you are a piece of the master.

As a woman, you have a different number of hormones than men. When applying these ancient healing strategies, there are special considerations for you. That's why I decided to dedicate an entire chapter to you. Once you complete Pillar 3, you can start on the strategies in this chapter. This chapter will provide a complete guide for how to use keto and fasting, whether you're a cycling woman or postmenopausal.* If you're in perimenopause, you can follow the program for cycling women. Let's start with the ladies who currently have a monthly cycle.

* I want to give credit where it's due for this research I'm about to share with you. Dr. Mindy Pelz, Dr. Stephanie Estima, Dr. Caitlin Czezowski, Dr. Carrie Jones, Dr. Sonya Jensen, Cynthia Thurlow, and Dr. Daniel Pompa have really helped me understand how to apply keto and fasting to women.

WHAT DOES YOUR PERIOD SAY ABOUT YOUR HEALTH?

On the *Metabolic Freedom* podcast, Dr. Stephanie Estima, author of *The Betty Body*, said, "Your monthly bleed is your hormonal report card."[1] Your menstrual cycle tells you about the hormonal status inside your body. If you have very heavy bleeding, heavy clotting, mood swings, bloating, or sleep disturbances, it's your body's way of telling you to pay attention. This is your body communicating with you. Symptoms are not the problem; they are feedback from your amazing body.

For women who are in their reproductive years, it's important to think about this hormonal milieu throughout the month. For simplicity's sake, we're going to break this up into seven-day cycles. First you want to track your monthly cycle. There are several apps you can use—Clue is a good one (visit https://helloclue.com).

Days 1–7

When you look at the first seven days of your monthly cycle—the bleed week—the hormonal landscape is as follows: Most hormones are taking a break. Estrogen, testosterone, luteinizing hormone, and progesterone are low. The one hormone that's elevated is follicule-stimulating hormone (FSH), and its job is to continue to develop the follicle to help the one lucky egg to be released this month. During this follicular phase (seven days), you're more resilient to macronutrient restriction. I suggest you follow a macronutrient approach of 70 percent fat, 25 percent protein, and 5 percent carbohydrates. This is the optimal time to do a one-meal-a-day approach or even an extended-block fast (three-plus days). Since progesterone is not around during this week, your appetite won't be stimulated. This makes it much easier to fast.

Days 8–14

The second week, which occurs just before ovulation, is the body's preparation phase for releasing an egg—whether or not pregnancy is the goal. During this time, estrogen becomes the rising star. Its concentration increases significantly from Week 1 to Week 2, signaling a shift into a more anabolic state that supports growth and repair. The primary role of this estrogen surge is to stimulate follicle development, setting the stage for successful ovulation. The other hormone that makes a debut is testosterone, which heightens your interest in sex and libido. This makes sense, because if you're having sex ahead of your ovulation, the chances increase of a sperm meeting the egg.

The number-one priority for the body is survival and reproduction. If your body prioritizes cortisol, it won't make progesterone efficiently. All fasts have a cortisol response via hormetic stress. This can be great during the first 14 days after the cycle, but not so good the 7 days leading up to the period (when your body needs to release progesterone to prepare your uterus for a possible pregnancy).

This is the best time to strength train. Building bone density and lean muscle mass is key for longevity in women. Resistance training would be terrific here in combination with protein. Protein stimulates the mechanistic target of rapamycin (mTOR), which is the opposite of autophagy, which you have learned is catabolic, as it breaks down and recycles damaged cell components. This is why I recommend you change your macros to the following: About 40 percent should come from fat, 45 percent should come from protein, and allows for a slight increase in carbohydrates, up to 15 percent. Your fasting schedule would shift to an 18/6 schedule, with two meals within your six-hour eating window.

Days 15–21

The third week occurs after ovulation, and the entire hormonal landscape changes once again. I suggest you return to the Week 1 guidelines: your macronutrient approach of 70 percent fat, 25 percent protein, and 5 percent carbohydrates. Now is when you want to be less restrictive with fasting, so that increased cortisol doesn't interfere with your progesterone production. Your fasting schedule changes to a 14/10 schedule with three meals during your 10-hour eating window.

The Magic of Resistant Starches

During Weeks 3 and 4, we see progesterone rise, which helps stimulate appetite and slow down your bowel movements. Consuming resistant starches during this time can be helpful. A resistant starch is a starch that resists digestion. The microbiota in the small intestine does not break them down. These starches enter the large intestine and become a food source for the microbiota in the large intestine. When you provide the large intestine with this fuel, it provides you with a gift called *butyrate*, a short-chain fatty acid. This helps with your sleep and cravings, and it assists in repairing the lining of your gut. The wonderful thing about resistant starches is that they don't technically count toward your carbohydrate intake—they are essentially "free" carbohydrates. Woohoo!

There are four main types of resistant starch—and each one works a little differently to feed your gut, balance blood sugar, and support fat-burning metabolism:

1. Type 1 is found in foods like beans, seeds, and whole grains, where the starch is physically trapped inside the fibrous cell walls, making it "resistant" to digestion.
2. Type 2 occurs naturally in raw potatoes, green bananas, and some tubers—these contain ungelatinized starch granules that resist enzymes until they're cooked.
3. Type 3 forms when certain starches are cooked and then cooled—think cold rice and potatoes. A process called retrogradation actually transforms digestible starch into resistant starch.
4. And finally, type 4 is man-made, created through chemical modification (you'll often find it in processed foods or supplements). While types 1 through 3 come straight from nature and nourish your microbiome, type 4 is more like the lab-grown cousin—not my first pick if you're after real metabolic benefits.

Here are Keto Flex–approved resistant starches:

- Green bananas
- Green-banana flour
- Green plantains
- Green-plantain flours

- Raw potatoes (you can grate a small amount of raw potato into a smoothie with lemon juice and cucumber)
- Raw potato starch
- Cold rice

The benefits of resistant starch include:

- **Reduction of insulin resistance.** Since resistant starch isn't digested, your insulin doesn't rise like with other starches that cause blood sugar problems.
- **Protection against colon cancer.** In a research study using mice, resistant starch killed precancerous cells in the gut and shrank cancerous lesions in the bowel.
- **Sleep improvement.** Resistant starch, which is a type of prebiotic, can also help you sleep better. A 2017 study found that rats fed prebiotics had better non-REM sleep (the restorative phase) than rats who weren't given prebiotics.[2]
- **Burning of fat and curbing of hunger.** Resistant starch can help you control your weight. One study found that adding resistant starch to meals can make you feel fuller quicker, causing you to eat fewer calories.[3] Another found that women who ate pancakes made with a resistant starch plus protein burned more fat after the meal than women who ate pancakes without resistant starch.[4]

Days 22–28

Now we move into the fourth week. The seven days before your period is showtime! Progesterone reaches its peak on Days 21 and 22. If you do blood work during this week, you'll see the following things reduced: blood glucose, amino acids, glutathione, lipids, and vitamin D. This is because your body is literally taking all of your substrates for energy and throwing it into your endometrium to thicken the lining and get you ready. I recommend more yoga, walks, and slowing down with your workouts during these seven days leading up to your period.

This is the best week to flex out of ketosis and increase your caloric load. I recommend the following macronutrient changes: 100–150 total grams of healthy carbohydrates, at least 100 grams of protein, less than 40 grams of fat, and no fasting. If you don't do this, you're going against your physiology, and Mother Nature always gets the last laugh (you may find yourself elbow deep in a bag of chips or a pint of ice cream).

My favorite carbohydrates for you at this time are squash, sweet potatoes, yams, yucca, citrus fruits, and ancient grains. You can find an entire list in Appendix B at the end of this book.

KETO FLEX FOR POSTMENOPAUSAL WOMEN

To the menopausal women: You are beautiful. You are not forgotten. Your wisdom and wrinkles are badges of honor. Let's discuss how keto and fasting applies to you.

When you're postmenopausal you can transfer all the energy that would be used building up the uterine lining every month for something else. These are your golden years, ladies!

As you move from later stages of perimenopause to postmenopause, you tend to become more insulin resistant. This means that your cells are not as sensitive to the effect of insulin, and it will have a harder time doing its job. Muscles also become resistant through anabolic resistance, and it takes more for muscle to grow. This is where we see testosterone, estrogen, and other hormones drop down, which can result in symptoms—you have to work harder to maintain what you have.

When you're over 40, you have an organ that is literally shutting down: the ovaries. There's no other time in your life that this happens unless you have an organ removed. The ovaries make estrogen, progesterone, and testosterone, and now this job is handed off to the adrenal glands and body fat.

A keto approach is wonderful here with the caveat of cyclical protein. Here's a 28-day protocol for postmenopausal women:

Weeks 1 and 2: Follow the 2/2/2/2 rule, hit protein requirements, consume less than 20 grams of total carbohydrates per day, and follow an 18/6 intermittent-fasting schedule. Having breakfast and lunch but skipping dinner works best. These two weeks are great to pair with strength training. This will help with new bone growth and breaking down old bone tissue to maintain muscle mass and bone density for longevity. My favorite exercises are squats, push-ups, shoulder presses, and walks with your dog.

Weeks 3 and 4: Follow the 5-1-1 rule:

- **5 days of intermittent fasting for 16 to 20 hours.** When you're eating during the 4-to-8-hour window, stick to a ketogenic (high healthy fats) approach. Keto macros = 80 percent fat, 15 percent protein, 5 percent carbohydrates.
- **1 24-hour water-only fast day** (dinner to dinner).
- **1 keto flex (feast) day.** Have three meals of high (healthy) carbohydrates and/or protein. Consume at least 150 grams of healthy carbs and/or protein. Eat less than 40 total grams of fat on this day.

Another thing to consider is that estrogen tends to decrease during menopause, and while you may no longer have this estrogen production from the ovaries, you can improve this through resistance training. Stress is an important component here, because after menopause your main source of estrogen will be from your adrenal glands, which also produce cortisol when you're stressed. The best way to prevent overwhelming your adrenal glands is to produce the hormone oxytocin, which is made in the hypothalamus and released into the bloodstream by the pituitary gland. Its main function is to facilitate childbirth, which is one of the reasons it's called the "love drug" or "love hormone." Oxytocin, like endorphins or serotonin, promotes positive feelings. Here are some easy ways to produce oxytocin:

- Gratitude journaling (I call gratitude "vitamin G")
- Laughter (funny movies, TV shows, and friends)
- Hugs (10 seconds or more for an oxytocin boost)
- Sex (orgasm helps with oxytocin)
- Favorite hobbies
- Snuggling pets

MENOPAUSE AND BONE LOSS

Preventing bone loss is an important concern for women on their menopause journey and during postmenopausal stages. Menopause significantly speeds up bone loss and increases the risk of osteoporosis. Research shows that women can lose up to 20 percent of their bone mass during the menopausal transition. Globally, approximately 1 in 10 women over the age of 60 currently have osteoporosis, while lifetime risk estimates suggest that up to 1 in 2 postmenopausal women will develop osteoporosis at some point, and most will suffer a fracture during their lifetime. Fractures (broken bones) cause pain and reduced mobility and function. Fractures are associated with decreased quality of life and increased mortality.

Estradiol is one of three estrogen hormones naturally produced in the body. The effects of lower estradiol are clearly seen in women experiencing menopause. During this process, women naturally have lower levels of estradiol as the ovaries no longer produce it, causing the menstrual cycles to stop. This change often causes mood swings, vaginal dryness, hot flashes, and night sweats—the symptoms commonly associated with menopause. Over time, lower estradiol levels can lead to osteoporosis. However, the Keto Flex lifestyle supports bone health by emphasizing high-quality protein and essential amino acids—the very building blocks your body uses to maintain strong, resilient bones and preserve lean muscle mass that protects your skeletal system.

Vitamin D and calcium also play a part in bone health. Vitamin D allows your body to absorb calcium, which is necessary for building strong, healthy bones. Without enough vitamin D and calcium, bones may not form properly in childhood and can lose mass, become weak, and break easily in adulthood. Even if you get enough calcium in your diet, your body will not absorb that calcium if you don't get enough vitamin D.

I recommend the following supplements for menopausal women to support bone health:

- Perfect Amino: 10 capsules per day
- Systemic Formulas DV3: 2 capsules per day with food (Once the bottle is done, take 30 days off.)
- Systemic Formulas CAL: 5 capsules per day with food (Once the bottle is done, take 30 days off.)

Each of these supplements plays a specific role in strengthening bones and supporting hormonal balance during menopause. Perfect Amino provides the eight essential amino acids in their most absorbable form, helping your body maintain lean muscle mass, repair tissues, and build the collagen matrix that gives bones their strength and flexibility. Systemic Formulas DV3 is a unique blend designed to enhance vitamin D_3 absorption and utilization, supporting calcium transport into the bones and optimizing hormonal pathways that protect against bone loss. Systemic Formulas CAL delivers bioavailable calcium along with synergistic cofactors like magnesium and trace minerals, ensuring that calcium actually reaches and strengthens bone tissue rather than depositing in soft tissues. Together, these three work in harmony to support bone density, muscle integrity, and overall metabolic health—especially vital for women transitioning through menopause when estrogen levels naturally decline. You can find all of these supplements, and more, over at benazadi.com.

▲▼▲

You may find that even though you're following this special protocol geared to your cycle, you're still having trouble and experiencing unwanted symptoms. In the next chapter, I'll share my top trouble-shooting tips for the most common symptoms that may arise.

CHAPTER TEN

KETO NINJA HACKS: EASY TIPS THAT MAKE KETO AND FASTING EFFORTLESS

When you make dietary and lifestyle changes, you may experience symptoms along the way. But symptoms are not a bad thing—they're a gift from your innate intelligence. Your body is always communicating with you.

John Miller came to me frustrated and discouraged. He had been "doing everything right" for years—following keto, watching his carbs—yet his body was still fighting him. The symptoms were loud: chronic knee pain, extreme fatigue, poor mobility, stubborn weight, and a sense that his body was working against him rather than with him.

Instead of ignoring those symptoms or trying to silence them, we treated them as feedback.

John's symptoms weren't a sign that his body was broken—they were signals that his metabolism needed a different conversation. Once we adjusted his approach to support fat adaptation, mineral balance, meal timing, movement, and stress, those signals began to change.

Within 30 days, John lost over 44 pounds. But more importantly, his pain eased, his energy improved, and everyday tasks that once felt impossible—climbing stairs, bending down, moving freely—became manageable again.

John didn't force his body into submission. He listened to it. And when he did, his symptoms transformed from obstacles into guideposts—pointing him toward healing.

After taking thousands of people through my four-pillar protocol, I've noticed the most common symptoms that occur, and I have solutions for each of them. This chapter is all about troubleshooting any keto and fasting symptoms you experience.

THE KETO FLU

In Chapter 5 I introduced the keto flu and my solution for it. But it's worth mentioning again, since it's common for keto beginners who don't transition properly. Calling it the keto flu gives keto a bad name. As I said earlier, we should call it "carbohydrate-withdrawal symptoms."

It's really quite simple. Carbohydrates are stored in the body with water. When you lower your carb intake, your body initially responds by excreting more water and retaining less. As you lose water, this may give you a quick "lean" look. Fewer carbs means less insulin release, causing the kidneys to release more sodium. This loss of sodium impacts the balance of other key electrolytes, potassium, and magnesium. These are minerals that carry an electrical charge. Vital for health and survival, they spark cell function throughout the body, support hydration, and help the body produce energy.

As carb intake decreases and electrolytes are increasingly excreted from the body in urine, imbalances of these electrolytes trigger the keto flu symptoms.[1] Keto flu symptoms typically include a headache, brain fog, fatigue, and an overall feeling of being unwell as your body transitions from burning sugar to burning fat for fuel. Ensuring adequate fluid and electrolyte intake can help counter some of these symptoms. This is why I developed the Keto Kamp Cocktail. Drink this every morning for at least seven days. You can also take high-quality electrolytes and minerals; my favorite brands are Beam Minerals, Redmond's, Upgraded Formulas, and Keto Chow.

KETO KAMP COCKTAIL

Servings: 1

16 ounces spring water
2 tablespoons apple cider vinegar
2 teaspoons cream of tartar (for extra potassium)
1 pinch high-quality salt

Mix together with a spoon, and drink first thing in the morning for 7 days.

KETO WITHOUT A GALLBLADDER

What does it mean if you don't have a gallbladder? Well, it means that you had it removed for some medical reason. The root-cause problem was likely never addressed, and the doctors just took it out. This could be because of gallstones related to cholesterol or an infection. Gallbladder removal is one of the top 10 procedures in the United States.

The gallbladder is there for a reason. Its job is to store your bile. As you may recall, bile is a digestive liquid that's produced in the liver and contains bile salts and other substances that help to break down fats from our diet. If you had your gallbladder removed, you can still benefit from ketosis! First, let's talk about the problems that can occur when you begin eating too many healthy fats. A great test to order from your doctor is the GGT test. If this is elevated, or your ALT, AST, or cholesterol is wonky, you most likely have very thick bile. This makes it difficult for your body to move the bile into the small intestine, which will result in an intolerance to fats. Symptoms may include:

- Gas
- Bloating
- Diarrhea
- Constipation
- Liver pain
- Loose, fatty stools

Here are the five steps to doing keto without a gallbladder:

Step #1: Eat smaller meals, and space out your fats for the first 14 days to allow the liver to adjust. Chew frequently to allow your body to produce digestive enzymes and stomach acid.

Step #2: Consume more fiber with your meals to slow the breakdown of fat. My favorite keto sources of fiber include:

- Avocados
- Pecans
- Steamed collard greens
- Cauliflower
- Broccoli
- Raw coconut

Step #3: Eat more bitter-rich foods to stimulate healthy bile flow. Bitter is better! Add these bitter-rich foods to your keto diet:

- Gingerroot/ginger tea
- Dandelion greens/tea
- Artichokes (bile builder/fiber)
- Coffee
- Lemons/limes
- Radishes
- Radicchio
- Cranberries
- Basil, thyme, rosemary (smell these to stimulate stomach enzymes)
- Cilantro and parsley
- Apple cider vinegar (thins bile)

Step #4: Consume medium-chain triglycerides (MCTs) because they bypass digestion, not requiring bile to break them down. My top five sources of MCTs (in order):

1. MCT oil (Start small with 1 teaspoon and build up to a maximum of 1 tablespoon.)
2. Organic, unrefined coconut oil (1 tablespoon daily)
3. Palm kernel oil (organic, unrefined, and sustainably sourced) (1 tablespoon daily)
4. Raw, grass-fed goat and sheep dairy (2 to 4 ounces daily)
5. Grass-fed butter or grass-fed ghee (1 tablespoon daily)

Step #5: Supplement the right way to support the liver as it adjusts to breaking down more fat on keto. I suggest you take the following supplements:

- Systemic Formulas D Digest: Take 2 capsules before each meal.
- Surthrival Herbal Digestive Bitters spray: Follow bottle instructions; take right before meals.

SLEEP ISSUES

Sleep challenges on keto are a temporary problem in which someone new to keto has difficulty falling or staying asleep. People who experience this usually do so within the first few days of reducing carbohydrates. Several things happen when you're starting keto, from having low glucose levels to possible electrolyte imbalances and digestive issues. These things can prevent you from getting quality sleep. While this is usually corrected within a few days, there are a few things you can do to speed up the process.

Raw Honey and MCT Oil Before Bed

During the night, your brain uses a lot of energy. One efficient form of brain energy comes from sugar stored in your liver, called liver glycogen. So, having a little extra sugar before bed can help your brain function better at night. You might think that honey is not keto friendly and will prevent you from burning fat and producing ketones, but if you take 1 tablespoon of MCT oil with the honey, you will produce enough ketones to remain in fat-burning mode.

Why raw honey? It has more beneficial nutrients than conventional honey, and rodent studies show raw honey may help you unwind. Take 1 to 2 teaspoons of raw honey before bed and see if it helps with your sleep. Keep in mind this is a short-term solution, not something you do long term.

Banana Tea Is Nature's Nyquil

Have you heard of banana tea before? I heard about it from Dr. Michael Breus. It turns out, the peel of the banana has more potassium and magnesium than the banana itself. Here's how you make it: Grab an entire organic banana. Leave the peel on but cut off the ends. Place it in a pot with 3 to 4 cups of water. Boil until the peel turns brown and then pour the water into a cup. This is keto friendly, and it does not break your fast.

SUGAR CRAVINGS

It's interesting—if I pulled out a cigarette in public and started smoking in front of people, most would look at me and think, *Dude, smoking kills.* But if I pulled out a candy bar and started eating it, they wouldn't have a second thought. But sugar kills just as many people as smoking does! Yet, we've been conditioned to believe that eating sugar is normal. Sugar has addictive properties, and animal studies show that its effects on the brain's reward system can resemble those of addictive drugs like cocaine.[2] As you make your transition from sugar burner to fat burner, you may notice sugar cravings flare up. If you have a real sugar addiction (like I used to have), I suggest working with a health practitioner who understands addiction. I'm also sharing a protocol that can work really well for sugar cravings on keto.

Glutamine

L-glutamine is an amino acid, which is a building-block protein necessary for blood sugar regulation. This amino acid is used as a supplement to help support the reduction of sugar cravings and also to increase gut health. L-glutamine is a fuel source for the cells in the small intestines, helping to achieve optimum intestinal health in the face of GI challenges. As a short-term supplement, L-glutamine can help to diminish normal sugar cravings. When blood sugar is low, glutamine quickly and easily converts to glucose, and studies have found it to be superior to pure glucose.[3]

When a craving hits for sugar or refined carbohydrates, L-glutamine can rapidly satiate this craving without decreasing insulin sensitivity. This means it can help you avoid reaching for less nutritious foods like candy, cookies, and cakes. L-glutamine calms the part of your brain that lights up when you experience a sugar/carb craving. Take 500 milligrams of L-glutamine powder, up to three times each day. Glutamine will help you wean.

Sleep!

When your sleep suffers, your blood sugars increase. Sleep deprivation can cause you to have the blood sugars of a type 2 diabetic. Yikes. Studies show that even one night of sleep deprivation disrupts key hunger hormones, increasing appetite. It also affects the way your brain's motivation centers respond to the sight or thought of food.[4] So, do your best to get enough rest!

KETO RASH

The keto rash is uncommon but can occur in some people following a low-carbohydrate approach. It's an itchy, red rash that occurs primarily on the upper back, chest, and abdomen. If you search Google, you'll see posts about this happening to people, with many theories as to why. The truth is that we don't have a specific cause, but I've seen improvements with my students when they implement the following tips:

- **Wipe off your sweat/take a shower.** The ketone body, acetone, can be irritating to the skin for some people, and the more you sweat while doing keto, the more it ignites the keto rash. A simple solution here is to wipe your sweat off quickly whenever sweating and to take a shower immediately after exercise.
- **Increase your protein intake.** Another tip that has worked, and I'm not exactly sure why, is increasing protein intake.

- **Add more bitters to your diet.** One more possible cause of the keto rash is a bile deficiency. I've written at length about the importance of healthy bile on keto, and it seems that some people who have thick bile tend to experience the keto rash. The solution is the bitters I spoke about on page 72. You might need additional liver support through ox bile supplementation, castor oil packs, coffee enemas, and/or taking extra liver support supplementation.
- **Increase your carbs.** If none of these tips work for you, then bringing your total carbohydrates up to 100 grams per day to get yourself out of ketosis should do the trick within one to two days. Then you can reenter and try again.

HIGH CHOLESTEROL AND LDL

This one is simple. It's usually not a problem when your cholesterol and LDL rise on keto. I know this is not what your doctor might tell you. You will feel much better with higher cholesterol and LDL levels, and your HDL should also increase, which is your body's janitorial system to clean out your arteries. You should also see a decline in triglycerides and in inflammatory markers, such as high-sensitivity C-reactive protein, homocysteine, and fasting insulin.

HEADACHES

The most common reason for headaches is a loss of electrolytes. Drink the Keto Kamp Cocktail (page 117) to help replenish your electrolytes. If you're already keeping up your electrolytes, then the other cause is high-histamine keto foods. Histamines are chemicals your immune system makes. They act like bouncers at a club, helping your body get rid of something that's bothering you—in this case, an allergy trigger, or *allergen*.

Histamines start the process that hustles those allergens out of your body or off your skin. They can make you sneeze, tear up, or itch—whatever it takes to get the job done. They are part of your body's defense system. If your headache is accompanied with the previously mentioned symptoms, then chances are you're sensitive to histamine foods. Try to limit the following common keto histamine foods:

- Packaged meat (deli meats)
- Aged cheeses (cheddar, gruyère, manchego, gouda, and parmesan)
- Fermented foods (sauerkraut, pickles, kimchi)
- Chocolate and cocoa
- Dried fruit
- Fermented dairy products, including cheese, yogurt, and buttermilk
- Alcohol
- Seafood (shell or fin fish; frozen, fresh, canned, or smoked)
- Spinach
- Spices, including curry powder, cayenne, chili, cloves, cinnamon, nutmeg
- Tea
- Tomatoes (fresh, canned, pureed, or in sauces)
- Vinegar and related products (for example, ketchup and mustard)
- Yeast

NAUSEA

The number-one cause of keto nausea is bile deficiency. Continue supporting your liver by eating the bitters we outlined earlier. Consider taking liver support and ox bile supplementation. If the problem persists, spread out your fats by eating more frequent, smaller keto meals until your liver adapts. This should take only a few days.

FATIGUE

When you first start a workout routine, you get sore. When you make the transition from sugar burner to fat burner, you might get "keto sore." What is keto sore? Symptoms can occur, and the most common one is fatigue. If your keto fatigue is happening within the first few days, then increase your minerals and electrolytes. As I explained earlier about the keto flu, as your body lowers insulin levels, the kidneys shed excess water weight along with minerals and electrolytes. You can double down on your electrolytes to see if this resolves the issue. Give it a few days as your body is still adapting to the new changes, and once it's an efficient fat burner, the fatigue will dissipate.

What if you're experiencing fatigue weeks into the protocol? This is more uncommon, but it can happen. I suggest revisiting—and optimizing—the fundamentals of health, sleep, stress, and movement. If you do, and you're still experiencing fatigue, then you can try exogenous (made outside of your body in supplement form) ketones. Ideally, we want your metabolism to produce ketones endogenously (within your body) as a by-product of fat burning. However, there's a time and place for exogenous ketone supplementation. There are three types of exogenous ketones: ketone salts, ketone esters, and butanediol (BDO).

Ketone salts won't be found in your table-side salt grinder. These supplements usually are found in powder form, which can be mixed with a liquid and consumed. Ketone salts are composed of a ketone body (usually BHB) bound to one of several minerals that may include sodium, potassium, calcium, or magnesium. Some salts also include an amino acid like lysine or arginine. The fact that ketones come bound to another mineral or amino acid makes ketone salts one way to consume ketones plus some necessary nutrients. But they aren't without certain considerations. A disadvantage is the possible side effects, often gastrointestinal issues. This may be a result of the acid load and/or mineral load that is obtained when consuming BHB salts at high doses.

Ketone esters are called acetoacetate diesters (1,3-butanediol acetoacetate diesters), and they consist of the ketone body acetoacetate and butanediol, connected by an ester bond (hence the name "ketone ester"). The AcAc diester produces a milder elevation in blood BHB (~1mM) compared to other ketone supplements.

As with some of the ketone salts, AcAc diester has been described as "unpalatable" and routinely produces GI symptoms in research participants who consume it. This and other potential side effects may lead to performance declines. I don't recommend using this ketone supplement prior to exercise, especially if it's your first time experimenting with it.

Butanediol, called R-1,3-butanediol (R-1,3-BDO), is another exogenous ketone that can be used to raise BHB levels. When consumed, R-1,3-BDO undergoes a series of oxidation steps in the liver. This exogenous ketone is converted into the physiological ketone bodies R-3-hydroxybutyrate and acetoacetate. Only 29–38 percent of R-1,3-butanediol uptake is accounted for by conversion into physiological ketone bodies.[5]

It has been shown in rats that a racemic BDO, or a mixture of chirally pure molecules, can raise blood BHB up to 1 mM.[6] Chirality refers to a property of certain molecules that exist in two mirror-image forms, often called left-handed and right-handed isomers. Although these forms share the same chemical formula, the body can metabolize them differently, sometimes using one form efficiently while the other is less active or follows a separate metabolic pathway. As a result, racemic mixtures—containing both forms—may produce variable biological effects compared with a single, chirally pure molecule. There are two other papers that examined the effects of BDO in human athletes. They found similar results where racemic BDO managed to consistently raise blood BHB up to 1 mM as well.[7]

I personally use and recommend the exogenous ketones from Real Ketones, KEY, Ketone-IQ, and Kenetik.

For the most part, exogenous ketones come in the form of BHB or acetoacetate. While the route to ketosis differs, the signaling effects of exogenous versus endogenous ketones are virtually the same—BHB and AcAc from the liver are no different structurally from BHB or

AcAc taken as a supplement. It's just simple biochemistry! However, if you take exogenous ketones without doing the work of rebuilding your metabolism to produce them endogenously, you will not get the same benefits at the end of the day. To rebuild your metabolism and produce ketones naturally, follow the Keto Flex approach, combining intermittent fasting, clean keto foods, and metabolic flexibility cycles that train your body to burn fat efficiently on its own.

Taking exogenous ketones daily can help with keto-related fatigue. They may also support mental clarity and help improve exercise performance. Exogenous ketones are intended to supplement—not replace—dietary and lifestyle changes.

MUSCLE CRAMPS

Muscle cramps are often a sign of decreased magnesium, and sometimes potassium. Cramping happens a lot, not just on keto. Magnesium is the focus. Here are some magnesium-rich foods:

- **Grass-fed beef:** a rich, bioavailable source of magnesium with virtually no antinutrients; also provides zinc and creatine for muscle and metabolic health
- **Avocados:** packed with magnesium, potassium, and healthy monounsaturated fats that support insulin sensitivity and hormone balance
- **Wild-caught salmon:** delivers magnesium plus omega-3 fatty acids that reduce inflammation and support mitochondrial health
- **Grass-fed cheese (like gouda or swiss):** provides magnesium, calcium, and vitamin K_2 in a highly absorbable form that supports bone and cardiovascular health

Keep in mind our soil is depleted and has less magnesium, so you may need to supplement.

Sodium is also a good idea, which you can find in your Keto Kamp Cocktail. Pickles and pickle juice can help too.

CONSTIPATION

Constipation is not fun. When you're backed up, your body can't efficiently eliminate toxins. Instead, these compounds—including estrogen that has already been used and marked for elimination—can be reabsorbed into circulation.

This is different from estrogen as a whole, which plays essential roles in metabolism, bone health, and brain function. The problem arises when metabolized estrogen meant to leave the body is recycled, increasing inflammatory and hormonal stress. Keto diet constipation is likely caused by one or more of the following factors:

- Your gut bacteria are taking time to adapt from a standard American diet to a diet higher in fat and protein.
- You have low stomach acid.
- Your bile production is lagging because your liver is sluggish.
- Your body is having a hard time processing the extra protein.
- You're chronically dehydrated.

The good news is that there are several things you can do to get things moving along. The first step is to make your stomach more acidic. You can easily do this by taking 1 to 2 tablespoons of apple cider vinegar before your meals and drinking water with lemon or lime. I also suggest avoiding the chronic use of alkaline water, as your gut needs to remain naturally acidic for proper digestion, nutrient absorption, and microbial balance.

Another option is to support the liver's ability to produce bile, which acts as a detergent to break down dietary fat. You can do this easily by eating more bitter-rich foods. We discussed this more in depth earlier in the book.

If you suspect it's a dehydration issue, then proper hydration is key. How much water should you drink? The old health dogma given out by practitioners is to drink half your body weight in ounces. I don't necessarily agree with this advice. Instead, I recommend looking at the color of your urine. You want your urine to be mostly clear, not completely clear or too yellow. If you're dehydrated, then drink natural spring water first thing in the morning with high-quality electrolytes.

Supplements can help too:

- **Magnesium** helps increase the amount of water in the intestines, which can help with bowel movements. It may be used as a laxative due to these properties, or as a supplement for magnesium deficiency. Taking 400 milligrams per day seems to work well.
- **Potassium** is needed in your colon walls to ensure that peristaltic action occurs. Without potassium, colon walls are weak and unable to respond and contract properly when fecal matter needs to be moved. Taking 400 milligrams of potassium per day is a good strategy.

We also need to consider your nervous system balance. Your nervous system has two main branches: the sympathetic branch, which is responsible for fight or flight, and the parasympathetic branch, which is responsible for rest, digestion, and elimination. When you're sympathetic dominant, the body is in a fight-or-flight, stressful state, and pooping is not the primary goal—survival is. Finding ways to balance your nervous system and achieve more parasympathetic activity can signal to your bowel that it's "safe" to eliminate. There are several things you can do to activate your parasympathetic nervous system. My favorite activities are gratitude journaling (vitamin G), nostril breathing instead of mouth breathing, walking in nature, and meditation.

Lastly, your eliminating position plays a role here. Are you sitting properly when you go to the bathroom? The closure mechanism of your gut is not designed in such a way to open properly when you're sitting normally. There's a muscle that encircles the gut when you're sitting or standing; this pulls it in one direction, creating a kink in the tube. This mechanism is an extra insurance policy in addition to the sphincters. When there's a kink, it's like your garden hose not properly releasing water, so you unbend it, and water flows freely and naturally. When you have a kink in your digestive system, your feces are blocked. The goal is relaxing your muscles so the poop is free to be released. Squatting has been the natural pooping position since the dawn of humankind. The modern sitting toilet has existed only since indoor sanitation became common in the late 1800s. Squatting makes pooping easier and faster in the following four ways:

1. **In the squatting position, gravity does most of the work.** The weight of the torso presses against the thighs and naturally compresses the colon. Gentle pressure from the diaphragm supplements the force of gravity.
2. **Squatting relaxes the puborectalis muscle**, allowing the anorectal angle to straighten and the bowel to empty completely.
3. **Squatting lifts the sigmoid colon to unlock the "kink" at the entrance to the rectum.** This kink also helps prevent incontinence by taking some of the pressure off the puborectalis muscle.
4. The colon is equipped with an inlet valve (the ileocecal valve) and an outlet valve (the puborectalis muscle). **Squatting simultaneously closes the inlet valve,** to keep waste from pushing back up into the small intestine, **and opens the outlet valve**, to allow waste to pass freely out of the body. The sitting position defeats the purpose of both valves, making elimination difficult and incomplete and increasing the risk of waste backing up into the small intestine where it should not be.

You don't have to risk getting caught by your neighbors pooping in your backyard. There are several products on the market that you place around your toilet that mimic this natural pooping position. The Squatty Potty is the most popular. (Each bathroom in my home has one.)

THE DAWN PHENOMENON (HIGH MORNING BLOOD SUGAR)

All mammals experience the dawn phenomenon (aka dawn effect) when they first wake up. Also called the Somogyi effect, this is a natural process that occurs in the morning. This happens for a couple of reasons.

First, your liver releases sugar from stored glycogen to bump up your blood sugar to give you a burst of energy to wake up in the morning. As you shift from an unconscious, sleepy state to starting your day, the body wants to prime you to get ready and move, like pushing the gas pedal on your car and revving your engine. This bump in glucose can also happen after you've taken a nap that's longer than 45 minutes.

The second cause of the dawn phenomenon is related to the hormone cortisol.[8] If you're waking up around sunrise, your body is naturally in sync with nature, and the light outside will signal to your adrenal glands to produce cortisol. This also helps with energy and kick-starts your day.[9] The cortisol impact on the dawn effect is secondary to the liver. Cortisol would delay the dawn effect, not necessarily cause it. As your blood sugar temporarily increases from these two processes, the pancreas should produce a pinch of insulin to remove the extra glucose from your bloodstream and shuttle it into your cells. This short-term blood glucose increase shouldn't be extraordinarily high and should last 30 minutes to 2 hours, until your body deals with it.

- Normal dawn effect glucose numbers: 85–100 mg/dL
- Abnormal dawn effect glucose numbers: 100 mg/dL lasting longer than 2 hours

If your dawn effect is higher than you'd like, and lasting several hours, there are a few reasons why. The hormone glucagon plays a role here. Your pancreas makes glucagon to help regulate your blood glucose (sugar) levels. Glucagon increases your blood sugar level and prevents it from dropping too low, whereas insulin decreases blood sugar levels. Glucagon gets released when the liver dumps sugar into the bloodstream in the morning, and then insulin should shut down the glucagon, but if you're insulin resistant, this may not happen, so you wind up with a big increase in your blood sugar that sticks around longer.

Growth hormone is another player here. Growth hormone is released during sleep, and this can also bump up glucose in the morning. If there's a strong cortisol response in the morning, another hormone called somatostatin is produced, which also blocks insulin.[10] Somatostatin is produced by many tissues in the body, principally in the nervous and digestive systems. This can cause high blood sugars throughout the day and potentially damage your tissues.

The best solution to an abnormal dawn phenomenon is to get a good night's sleep. When you improve your sleep, you'll be able to produce more growth hormone and less somatostatin. A simple strategy for better sleep, and to fix abnormal dawn effect readings, is to give yourself at least three hours of fasting before bed—even better if this is five hours. I have seen anecdotally with my students who have abnormal dawn effect readings that simply having them fast for five hours before bed fixes this issue. This means if you go to bed at 11 P.M., the kitchen should be closed by 6 P.M. at the latest.

The overall goal is to reverse insulin resistance and type 2 diabetes, which is the upstream cause of abnormal dawn effect levels.

WHAT TO DO IF YOU CAN'T GET INTO KETOSIS

Some people have trouble getting into ketosis. If you're one of these people, don't give up! I've found there are typically five reasons why you can't get into ketosis—and I have solutions for each one.

1. Too Many Carbohydrates

In general, most people can achieve ketosis by dropping their total carbohydrates to 50 grams per day. Others might need to be more restrictive—usually those who have been sugar burners for a long time. The solution is to drop your carbohydrates to below 20 grams per day. This isn't a long-term solution, but it can force your body to choose fat. Keep an eye out for "carbohydrate creep"!

2. Your Metabolism Needs More Time to Adapt

If you've been a sugar burner for several years, it may take you longer than a week to burn fat and produce ketones. This is completely normal. Patience truly is a keto virtue here. While most people who complete Pillar 1 will be in fat-burning mode, some people, especially those who have high insulin levels and/or diabetes, need more time. Continue working your way through the pillars, and it's only a matter of time before you achieve fat-burning ketosis. You can also stay in Pillar 1 an extra week or two if you'd like. Exogenous ketones can help "prime the pump" too. While I don't like to rely on exogenous ketones without doing the work, there is a time and place for them.

3. Too Much Fasting, Too Soon

You might be fasting too much, too soon. Fasting is a muscle you want to develop over time. When your body is metabolically inflexible, your brain is dependent on glucose in the form of carbohydrate calories. When you practice fasting before developing metabolic flexibility, it can be a struggle. When glucose gets low in the brain, the brain will send the body intense cravings for carbohydrates (sugar!) to fulfill its desire for glucose. You may have the willpower to persevere, but your innate intelligence will win this battle because it will start to raise cortisol and glucose, and even break down healthy protein to convert into sugar via gluconeogenesis to meet the brain's demand for glucose. Once your body is metabolically flexible, ketones come to the rescue so that the brain does not panic, cravings go away, and you feel optimal throughout the fast.

The solution is to shorten your fasting window as you build up your metabolic machinery. Keep working on your fat adaptation by following the 2/2/2/2 rule, drop total carbohydrates further (if needed), and then retry by expanding your fasting window hour by hour each day to see how your body (and brain) responds. A pro tip I teach my students is to track blood glucose and ketones during your fast. The trend you want to see is blood glucose gradually dropping while blood ketones are gradually increasing. If you see the opposite trend, it's time to break the fast and try again sometime soon.

Another great metric to see if fasting is working for you or against you is heart rate variability. Find your baseline, and work on increasing HRV. If you see your HRV drop, and it was a longer-than-usual fasting day, this could signal that your fast was too stressful on the body. I personally use the Oura ring to track my HRV during sleep.

4. Poor Sleep and/or Too Much Stress

Yes, too much stress will kick you out of ketosis. When cortisol is high, glucose follows, and ketones drop. There was a recent study in *Scientific American* that showed poor sleep produces higher levels of the stress hormone cortisol, higher levels of glucose, and higher levels of the hunger hormone ghrelin.[11] The solution is to practice one or more of these simple ways to reduce stress:

- Remember to practice gratitude journaling—what I call vitamin G.
- Practice self-love.
- Practice loving others.
- Get rid of toxic relationships!
- Turn off the news!
- Don't neglect your sleep.

Sleep is foundational for achieving perfect health. The topic of sleep is outside the scope of this book, but I recommend the following sleep experts to learn more: Devin Burke, Mollie Eastman, Matthew Walker, and Dr. Michael Breus.

5. Toxins

This is the most common reason why people struggle to get into ketosis, or why they keep getting kicked out of ketosis. We live in the most toxic world in the history of humanity. The number-one priority for the body is survival. When toxins enter the body via breathing, skin absorption, and eating, the body does not want these toxins to enter vital organs, which can potentially kill you. This is why peroxisome proliferator-activated receptor gamma (PPARγ) gets activated in the body as a survival mechanism. PPARγ takes those toxins and shuttles them into fat cells and can even create new fat cells for these toxins to live in. This is how toxins make you fat. Why is the body so cruel? It's trying to save your life! The body will do everything possible to survive in the moment, even if that means increasing chances of disease in the future by storing these toxins.

When you start your Keto Flex lifestyle, you will be shrinking and burning fat cells. The body can burn fat cells, but it can't burn toxins, so they get dumped into the bloodstream and reabsorbed. This can lead to not feeling well and also cellular membrane inflammation. When the membrane is inflamed, insulin will have a challenge delivering glucose into the cell and keeping glucose levels optimal in the bloodstream. The result could be higher glucose and lowered ketones.

The first step is to remove the interference. It doesn't really help to detox if you keep retoxing. Do an audit on your environment and remove toxins. Say no to cash register receipts. Many thermal paper receipts are coated with bisphenol A (BPA) or similar compounds. BPA can be absorbed through the skin and acts as an endocrine disruptor, meaning it can interfere with hormone signaling—especially estrogen metabolism. Limiting contact with receipts, declining them when possible, or washing your hands after handling them is a simple way to reduce unnecessary chemical exposure. Check your home for mold, drink out of glass bottles, stop microwaving plastic Tupperware, and speak with a biological dentist about your silver amalgam fillings.

The next step is to keep your downstream detoxification pathways open. This consists of your digestive system, lymphatic system, liver, kidney, and colon. Stay consistent with your bitters we spoke about earlier, as this does have a detoxification effect. You can also do the following for downstream detox support:

- Weekly massages (deep tissue and lymphatic)
- Dry brushing
- Trampoline jumping
- Daily movement
- Weekly chiropractic adjustments
- Red-light therapy
- Infrared sauna
- Foam rolling
- Morning stretching/yoga
- Proper supplementation

5 WAYS TO RAISE KETONES

The following tips have been scientifically proven to help you produce ketones:

Tip 1: Try caprylic acid. The medium-chain triglyceride (MCT) caprylic acid (C8) increases plasma ketone response more than coconut oil or other medium-chain triglycerides. Coconut oil naturally contains several different medium-chain fatty acids with varying carbon chain lengths, including caprylic acid (C8), capric acid (C10), and lauric acid (C12). When coconut oil is fractionated, specific fatty acids—such as caprylic acid—are isolated and concentrated. As a result, pure C8 oil delivers a much higher proportion of caprylic acid than whole coconut oil, which contains relatively less C8 because other fatty acid chains are still present. Take 1 to 2 tablespoons of caprylic acid in the morning.

Tip 2: Drink coffee. Great news, fellow coffee and tea drinkers: Caffeine has been shown to help with ketone production. Studies suggest caffeine intake increases plasma ketones! One study aimed to evaluate the acute ketogenic effect of two doses of caffeine in 10 healthy adults. Caffeine given at breakfast significantly stimulated ketone production in a dose-dependent manner and also raised plasma free fatty acids.[12] Drink 16 ounces of coffee (or tea) 90 minutes after waking up. Bonus points if you add the C8 oil to it!

Tip 3: Swap out all cow dairy for sheep and goat dairy. At some point, approximately 75 percent of the world's population loses the ability to process cow dairy.[13] Sheep and goat dairy are not only easier to digest, but also they contain 30 percent medium-chain triglycerides, which help your body produce ketones.

Tip 4: Supplement with L-carnitine. Carnitine is a substance that helps the body turn fat into energy. Think of L-carnitine as a shuttle bus delivering fatty acids to your mitochondria for ketone use! Studies suggest L-carnitine can help the process of fat utilization and insulin sensitivity.[14]

Tip 5: Sleep. You can't skip the fundamentals. If your sleep is poor, you'll have higher levels of cortisol the next morning. What follows cortisol? Glucose. And when glucose rises, ketones fall.

▲▼▲

Hopefully these ninja hacks have made your reset easier. In the final chapter, I'll make keto flexing even more effortless with some simple, delicious recipes that will satisfy your hunger—and your taste buds!

CHAPTER ELEVEN

FROM KITCHEN TO KETOSIS: TRANSFORMATIVE KETO FLEX RECIPES

The Keto Flex Reset doesn't mean you deprive your taste buds and count every calorie that goes into your body. The easiest way to adopt this new, healthy lifestyle is to follow the recipes I've outlined for you. These recipes meet my strict "clean keto" guidelines, focus on protein, and make sure you enter the fat-burning state of ketosis without having to rely on willpower. Below are some amazing recipes that will excite your taste buds and your hormones.

BUFFALO CHICKEN EGG MUFFINS

Hot sauce, chicken, and chives give these egg muffins a buffalo chicken vibe that is indulgent and delicious! You can cook the chicken for the muffins yourself if you like, but for extra ease, consider buying a prepared rotisserie chicken from the grocery store instead.

Servings: 2

- Prep Time: 10 minutes
- Cook Time: 25 to 30 minutes
- Total Time: 35 to 40 minutes

3 tablespoons butter, melted
6 large eggs
¼ teaspoon sea salt
¼ teaspoon ground black pepper
4 ounces chopped or shredded cooked chicken
2 tablespoons sugar-free hot sauce
2 teaspoons sliced chives

Preheat the oven to 375°F (190°C). Grease six muffin cups of a muffin tin with the butter.

Whisk the eggs with the salt and pepper until combined. Divide the chicken between the muffin cups and pour the eggs on top, ensuring there is an even amount in each one. Place the muffin tin on a baking sheet.

Bake the muffins until set and cooked through, about 25 to 30 minutes.

Remove the muffins from the pan and divide them between two plates.

Garnish them with the hot sauce and chives, and serve immediately.

Macros
Fat: 34 gram
Protein: 35.5 grams
Carbs: 1.5 grams

ASIAN-INSPIRED BEEF LETTUCE WRAPS

These flavorful wraps will leave you wanting more with the traditional Asian flavors of tamari, sesame, and cilantro. If you like, feel free to scale up the steak mixture so that you can quickly reheat throughout the week to stuff into buttery lettuce for lunch. A little sriracha makes for a delicious addition to these wraps!

Servings: 2

- Prep Time: 15 minutes, plus 30 minutes marinating time
- Cook Time: 3 to 5 minutes
- Total Time: 48 to 50 minutes

10 ounces flank or sirloin steak
2 tablespoons tamari
4 tablespoons sesame oil
1 tablespoon apple cider vinegar
2 teaspoons finely minced ginger
3 garlic cloves, minced
½ teaspoon sea salt
¼ teaspoon ground black pepper
8 Bibb or Boston lettuce leaves
2 tablespoons chopped cilantro

Thinly slice the steak into strips against the grain.

In a bowl, whisk the tamari with the sesame oil, vinegar, ginger, garlic, salt, and pepper until combined. Add the steak to the bowl and allow it to marinate for at least 30 minutes.

Heat a large skillet over medium-high heat. Add the steak mixture to the skillet and cook until the steak is just cooked through, about 3 to 5 minutes.

Divide the steak between the lettuce leaves and garnish them with cilantro.

Macros
Fat: 39.5 grams
Protein: 33.5 grams
Carbs: 4.5 grams

THAI-INSPIRED RED COCONUT CURRY CHICKEN SOUP

This Thai red curry with chicken and vibrant-green broccoli is warming, fragrant, and a little spicy. Bone-in chicken is often cheaper than chicken breasts, and it will stay juicy even if you end up cooking it a little longer.

Servings: 2

- Prep Time: 10 minutes
- Cook Time: 39 to 41 minutes
- Total Time: 49 to 51 minutes

4 tablespoons butter
4 chicken drumsticks
Sea salt and ground black pepper, to taste
3 tablespoons red Thai curry paste
1 cup coconut milk
1 cup chicken bone broth
1 cup broccoli florets
1 tablespoon chopped cilantro

Heat the butter in a large pot over medium heat. Season the chicken with salt and pepper to taste. Add the chicken to the pot and cook until golden on both sides, about 8 to 10 minutes. Remove the chicken from the pot and set aside.

Add the curry paste to the skillet and cook until fragrant, about 30 seconds. Stir in the coconut milk and chicken broth, and bring to a simmer.

Nestle the chicken into the coconut milk, cover, and simmer until cooked through, about 20 minutes.

Add the broccoli and cook until tender, about 10 minutes.

Divide the curry between two bowls, garnish with the cilantro, and serve immediately.

Macros

Fat: 45 grams

Protein: 46.5 grams

Carbs: 9.5 grams

LEMON-HERB CHICKEN WINGS

Lemony and herbaceous, these chicken wings are sure to be a hit. They include a combination of lemon zest and juice, ensuring they get both the fragrance and tanginess of the lemon.

Servings: 2

- Prep Time: 10 minutes
- Cook Time: 40 to 45 minutes
- Total Time: 50 to 55 minutes

8 chicken wings, split into flats and drumettes
2 tablespoons melted butter
1 tablespoon lemon zest
1 tablespoon freshly squeezed lemon juice
2 teaspoons Italian seasoning
½ teaspoon sea salt
¼ teaspoon ground black pepper

Preheat the oven to 400°F (205°C) and line a large baking sheet with parchment paper.

Toss the chicken wings with the remaining ingredients, until combined. Arrange the wings on the large baking sheet. Bake on the center rack of the oven for 20 minutes; turn the chicken wings and bake them until they are golden and cooked through, about another 20 to 25 minutes.

Divide the wings between two plates and serve immediately.

Macros
Fat: 37 grams
Protein: 36 grams
Carbs: 2 grams

GINGER-TAMARI BEEF WITH SHIRATAKI RICE

Tender steak is made even more succulent with fresh ginger, garlic, tamari, and hot sauce. Serving it with shirataki rice ensures you have something that can soak up the flavorful sauce.

Servings: 2

- Prep Time: 10 minutes, plus 30 minutes marinating time
- Cook Time: 3 to 5 minutes
- Total Time: 43 to 45 minutes

12 ounces sirloin steak, sliced into thin strips
6 tablespoons olive oil
2 tablespoons tamari
1 tablespoon apple cider vinegar
1 teaspoon ginger, finely grated
1 teaspoon Asian-style hot sauce such as sriracha, or more to taste
1 garlic clove, minced
Sea salt and ground black pepper, to taste
2 7-ounce packages shirataki rice
2 tablespoons finely chopped cilantro

Combine the steak with the olive oil, tamari, apple cider vinegar, ginger, sriracha, garlic, and salt and pepper to taste until combined. Marinate in the fridge for at least 30 minutes.

Heat a large nonstick skillet over medium-high heat. Add the steak and cook for 3 to 5 minutes, or until the steak is cooked to your desired doneness.

Cook the shirataki rice according to the package instructions.

Divide the rice between two bowls, top with the steak mixture, and garnish with cilantro before serving.

Macros

Fat: 48.5 grams

Protein: 38 grams

Carbs: 5.5 grams

THAI-INSPIRED BEEF SALAD (KETO FLEX)

This fresh-tasting salad has lots of fresh herbs and includes a tangy dressing with the brightness of lime. Flank steak is ideal here, as it is extremely high protein while being more lean than other cuts of beef.

Servings: 2

- Prep Time: 20 minutes, plus 30 minutes marinating time
- Cook Time: 8 minutes
- Total Time: 58 minutes

For the Steak

6 ounces flank steak

3 tablespoons tamari

¾ teaspoon sea salt

¼ teaspoon ground black pepper

For the Salad

24 cups chopped romaine or green leaf lettuce
4 red, orange, yellow, or green bell peppers, thinly sliced
4 English cucumbers, sliced into half moons
1 cup torn mint leaves
1 cup torn cilantro leaves
2 Thai chili peppers, thinly sliced

For the Dressing

6 tablespoons freshly squeezed lime juice
2 tablespoons tamari
1 teaspoon olive oil
2 garlic cloves, minced
¼ teaspoon red pepper flakes, or more to taste
¼ teaspoon sea salt
¼ teaspoon ground black pepper

Rub the steak with the tamari, salt, and pepper. Put it on a plate and allow it to marinate in the fridge for at least 30 minutes.

Heat a skillet over medium heat. Add the steak and cook it until medium rare, about 4 minutes per side or to desired doneness. Remove it from the heat and allow it to rest for at least 5 minutes before slicing it.

Meanwhile, for the salad, toss the lettuce with the remaining ingredients until combined.

For the dressing, in a bowl whisk all the ingredients until combined.

Toss the salad with the steak and dressing, divide it between two plates, and serve immediately.

Macros
Fat: 8.5 grams
Protein: 33 grams
Carbs: 51 grams

CRISPY LEMON-GARLIC CHICKEN THIGHS

Servings: 1

1 tablespoon ghee
1 bone-in chicken thigh
½ teaspoon sea salt
¼ teaspoon ground black pepper
½ teaspoon dried rosemary
2 garlic cloves, minced
Juice of ½ lemon

Preheat the oven to 400°F (205°C).

Heat the ghee in a cast-iron skillet over medium-high heat.

Pat the chicken thigh dry and season with salt, pepper, and rosemary.

Place the thigh skin-side down in the hot pan. Sear 5 to 6 minutes until golden and crispy.

Flip the chicken. Add the garlic and lemon juice to the pan.

Transfer the skillet to the oven and bake 15 to 18 minutes or until fully cooked.

Spoon the pan juices over the chicken before serving.

Macros

Fat: 28 grams

Protein: 32 grams

Carbs: 3 grams

STEAK AND EGGS POWER PLATE

A classic keto breakfast that stabilizes blood sugar and boosts fat burning.

Servings: 1

1 tablespoon butter
1 6-ounce grass-fed rib eye steak
Sea salt and ground black pepper, to taste
2 pasture-raised eggs

Heat a skillet on high and melt the butter in it.

Season the rib eye with salt and pepper.

Sear the steak 3 to 4 minutes per side for medium-rare.

Remove the steak and cook the eggs sunny-side up in the same pan.

Plate the steak with the eggs and spoon the remaining butter over the top.

Macros
Fat: 38 grams
Protein: 45 grams
Carbs: 1 gram

OLIVE OIL–POACHED SALMON

Silky, delicate salmon infused with citrus and herbs.

Servings: 1

¼ cup high polyphenol extra-virgin olive oil
1 garlic clove
1 sprig thyme
1 strip lemon peel
1 5-ounce wild salmon fillet
¼ teaspoon sea salt

Add the olive oil to a small pot over low heat.

Once the oil is warm, add the garlic, thyme, lemon peel, and salt to the pot.

Slide in the salmon and poach gently for 12 to 14 minutes.

Remove the fish with a spatula and spoon the infused oil over the top.

Macros
Fat: 36 grams
Protein: 34 grams
Carbs: 1 gram

BEEF AND CABBAGE BREAKFAST HASH

A low-oxalate, high-protein morning skillet.

Servings: 1

1 tablespoon beef tallow
5 ounces ground beef
½ cup shredded green cabbage
¼ cup diced zucchini
½ teaspoon smoked paprika
Sea salt, to taste

Heat the tallow in a skillet over medium heat.

Add the beef and brown it fully.

Add the cabbage, zucchini, and paprika.

Cook until the vegetables soften and their edges are crisp.

Season with salt and serve.

Macros
Fat: 30 grams
Protein: 36 grams
Carbs: 7 grams

GINGER-SESAME SALMON

A flavorful, Asian-inspired dish without soy or seed oils.

Servings: 1

1 tablespoon toasted sesame oil
1 garlic clove, minced
1 teaspoon ginger, grated
1 teaspoon coconut aminos
1 6-ounce wild salmon fillet
Sea salt, to taste

Preheat the oven to 375°F (190°C). Line a small baking sheet with parchment paper.

Mix the sesame oil, garlic, ginger, coconut aminos, and sea salt.

Place the salmon on the baking sheet and coat with the mixture.

Bake 12 to 15 minutes until flaky.

Macros
Fat: 28 grams
Protein: 35 grams
Carbs: 4 grams

CREAMY GARLIC SHRIMP BOWL

Rich, satisfying, and gut friendly.

Servings: 1

1 tablespoon butter
6 ounces wild shrimp
2 garlic cloves, minced
2 tablespoon heavy cream
¼ cup shredded cabbage
Sea salt and ground black pepper, to taste

Melt the butter in a pan.

Add the shrimp and sauté for 2 to 3 minutes, until pink.

Add the garlic and cook for 30 seconds.

Add the cream, salt, and pepper and simmer for 2 to 3 minutes.

Serve over the shredded cabbage.

Macros
Fat: 26 grams
Protein: 30 grams
Carbs: 5 grams

TALLOW-FRIED BURGERS WITH CARAMELIZED ONIONS

A carnivore-leaning, ultra-satisfying meal.

Servings: 1

1 tablespoon tallow
2 3-to-4-ounce ground beef patties
Sea salt and ground black pepper, to taste
¼ red or yellow onion, thinly sliced

Melt the tallow in a skillet.

Add the patties, season them with salt and pepper, and cook them for 3 to 4 minutes per side.

Remove the patties and add the onions to the same pan.

Cook until deeply browned.

Serve the burgers topped with the onions.

Macros
Fat: 34 grams
Protein: 40 grams
Carbs: 6 grams

CHILI-LIME CHICKEN SKILLET

Fast, bright, and fat burning.

Servings: 1

1 tablespoon ghee
1 6-ounce chicken breast
1 teaspoon chili powder
Sea salt, to taste
1 lime

Heat the ghee over medium-high heat.

Season the chicken with chili powder and salt.

Sear for 4 to 5 minutes per side.

Squeeze the lime's juice into the pan to finish.

Macros
Fat: 14 grams
Protein: 35 grams
Carbs: 4 grams

ZOODLE ALFREDO WITH GRILLED CHICKEN

Creamy comfort food under 10 carbs.

Servings: 1

1 5-ounce chicken breast
1 tablespoon butter
2 tablespoons heavy cream
2 tablespoons grated parmesan
1 small zucchini, spiralized
Sea salt and ground black pepper, to taste

Grill or pan-cook the chicken breast.

In a pan, melt the butter. Add the cream, salt, and pepper, and simmer lightly.

Add the parmesan. Stir until thickened.

Add the zoodles and toss for 30 to 60 seconds (don't overcook).

Slice the chicken and place on top of the zoodles.

Macros
Fat: 24 grams
Protein: 40 grams
Carbs: 8 grams

CRISPY DUCK BREAST WITH ROSEMARY DRIZZLE

High-fat gourmet simplicity.

Servings: 1

1 duck breast
1 sprig rosemary
Sea salt, to taste

Score the duck fat without cutting into the meat.

Place the skin-side down in a cold skillet.

Turn the heat to medium and render the fat for 6 to 8 minutes.

Flip and cook for 3 to 4 minutes more.

Spoon the rendered fat over the top and add the rosemary and salt.

Macros
Fat: 42 grams
Protein: 30 grams
Carbs: 0 grams

BISON RIB EYE WITH GARLIC BUTTER

Lean but deeply flavorful.

Servings: 1

1 6-ounce bison rib eye
Sea salt and ground black pepper, to taste
1 tablespoon butter
1 garlic clove, minced

Season the steak well with salt and pepper.

Heat a pan to high and sear the steak for 3 to 4 minutes per side.

Melt the butter with the garlic and pour over the steak.

Macros
Fat: 30 grams
Protein: 42 grams
Carbs: 1 gram

TURKEY PATTIES WITH LEMON CABBAGE SLAW

Light, refreshing, blood-sugar friendly.

Servings: 1

5 ounces ground turkey
1 cup shredded cabbage
Juice of 1/2 lemon
1 tablespoon extra-virgin olive oil
Sea salt and ground black pepper, to taste

Form the turkey into 2 patties.

Pan-fry for 4 to 5 minutes per side.

Toss the cabbage with the lemon, olive oil, and salt and pepper.

Serve the patties over the cabbage slaw.

Macros
Fat: 18 grams
Protein: 35 grams
Carbs: 7 grams

CREAMY COCONUT CHICKEN CURRY

Warm, anti-inflammatory, comfort forward.

Servings: 1

1 6-ounce chicken thigh
½ teaspoon turmeric
½ teaspoon ginger
1 garlic clove, minced
Sea salt
¼ cup coconut milk

Dice the chicken into chunks and brown them in the skillet.

Add the spices and garlic; sauté for 30 seconds.

Add the coconut milk and simmer for 8 to 10 minutes.

Macros
Fat: 28 grams
Protein: 32 grams
Carbs: 6 grams

SARDINE CITRUS BOWL

Simple, nutrient-dense, metabolic gold.

Servings: 1

1 can water-packed sardines
1 tablespoon extra-virgin olive oil
Juice of ½ lemon
Sea salt, to taste

Drain the sardines.

Plate them and drizzle the olive oil and lemon on the fish.

Add salt to taste.

Macros
Fat: 20 grams
Protein: 32 grams
Carbs: 0 grams

TALLOW-SEARED LAMB CHOPS

Rich, savory, mineral dense.

Servings: 1

1 tablespoon tallow
2 to 3 small lamb chops (6 ounces total)
Garlic powder
Sea salt, to taste

Heat the tallow on medium-high heat.

Add the lamb chops, garlic powder, and sea salt.

Sear the chops for 3 minutes per side.

Rest for 3 minutes before serving.

Macros
Fat: 34 grams
Protein: 38 grams
Carbs: 0 grams

CHILI-LIME SHRIMP LETTUCE CUPS

Fresh, bright, and perfect for summer.

Servings: 1

1 tablespoon butter
6 ounces shrimp
1 teaspoon chili powder
Juice of 1 lime
4 to 6 Bibb lettuce leaves

Melt the butter in a skillet.

Add the shrimp and chili powder.

Cook for 2 to 3 minutes on each side.

Add the lime juice, then fill the lettuce cups with the seasoned shrimp.

Macros
Fat: 18 grams
Protein: 32 grams
Carbs: 4 grams

KETO EGG DROP SOUP

A gut-healing, high-protein warm meal.

Servings: 1

2 cups bone broth
3 eggs
1 tablespoon butter
1 scallion, sliced
Sea salt, to taste

Bring the broth to a boil.

Lower the heat to a simmer.

Whisk the eggs in a bowl.

While stirring the broth, slowly drizzle the eggs into it.

Add the butter, scallions, and salt to taste.

Macros
Fat: 22 grams
Protein: 30 grams
Carbs: 4 grams

CRISPY PORK BELLY BITES

One of the easiest high-fat keto meals.

Servings: 1

6 ounces pork belly
½ teaspoon sea salt
½ teaspoon smoked paprika

Preheat the oven to 425°F (220°C).

Cut the pork belly into cubes.

Season with salt and paprika.

Roast for 30 to 35 minutes, flipping halfway through.

Macros
Fat: 44 grams
Protein: 34 grams
Carbs: 0 grams

GARLIC-GHEE SALMON FILLET

Fast, clean, blood-sugar stable.

Servings: 1

1 tablespoon ghee
2 garlic cloves, minced
1 6-ounce wild salmon fillet
Sea salt, to taste

Melt the ghee in a skillet.

Add the garlic and sea salt. Sauté for 30 seconds.

Add the salmon and cook for 4 to 5 minutes per side.

Spoon the garlic ghee over the fish.

Macros
Fat: 26 grams
Protein: 36 grams
Carbs: 1 gram

HERB-BUTTER TURKEY CUTLETS

Lean protein elevated by rich fats.

Servings: 1

1 6-ounce turkey cutlet
Sea salt, to taste
1 tablespoon butter
1 garlic clove, minced
½ teaspoon thyme

Season the turkey with salt.

Heat a skillet over medium heat and add the butter. Let it melt completely and gently foam, swirling the pan to coat the surface evenly.

Cook for 3 to 4 minutes per side in butter.

Add the garlic and thyme to finish.

Macros
Fat: 18 grams
Protein: 32 grams
Carbs: 2 grams

CAULIFLOWER FRIED RICE (BEEF EDITION)

A low-carb version of takeout comfort.

Servings: 1

1 tablespoon tallow
4 ounces ground beef
½ cup cauliflower rice
1 garlic clove, minced
1 egg
Sea salt, to taste

Heat the tallow in a skillet.

Add the beef and brown it fully.

Add the cauliflower rice and garlic; cook for 4 minutes.

Push the mixture aside. Scramble the egg in the pan.

Mix together and season with sea salt.

Macros
Fat: 28 grams
Protein: 35 grams
Carbs: 8 grams

KETO FLEX DAY RECIPES. HIGH CARB AND PROTEIN, LOW FAT. FOR FEAST DAYS.

CHICKEN AND SWEET POTATO POWER BOWL

High-protein, high-carb meal perfect after a tough training day.

Servings: 1

1 cup sweet potato cubes
1 6-ounce chicken breast
½ cup green beans
½ lemon
Sea salt and paprika, to taste

Roast the sweet potato cubes at 400°F (205°C) for about 25 minutes until soft.

Grill or bake the chicken breast until fully cooked.

Steam the green beans.

Assemble the vegetables and chicken in a bowl and squeeze the lemon's juice on top.

Season with salt and paprika.

Macros

Fat: 4 grams

Protein: 42 grams

Carbs: 54 grams

LEAN TURKEY AND RICE BOWL

Ultra-lean, clean-burning carb replenishment.

Servings: 1

6 ounces 99% lean ground turkey
½ cup diced carrots
1 tablespoon coconut aminos
Ground black pepper, to taste
1 cup cooked white rice

Lightly brown the turkey in a nonstick skillet (with no added fat).

Add the carrots and cook until soft.

Add the coconut aminos and black pepper.

Fold in the white rice and heat through.

Macros
Fat: 4 grams
Protein: 37 grams
Carbs: 56 grams

HIGH-PROTEIN BERRY RICE BREAKFAST

A clean, whole-food carb-up breakfast.

Servings: 1

3 egg whites
¾ cup cooked white rice
1 cup mixed berries (blueberries, raspberries, strawberries)
Cinnamon
1 teaspoon raw honey (optional)

Scramble the egg whites in a nonstick pan (with no added fat).

In a separate pot, warm the rice and mix it with the berries and cinnamon.

Add honey if desired.

Serve the egg whites on the side or mixed in.

Macros
Fat: 1 gram
Protein: 32 grams
Carbs: 52 grams

LEAN BEEF AND POTATO HASH

Perfect flex-day comfort meal.

Servings: 1

1 medium white potato, diced
5 ounces 96% lean ground beef
½ cup diced red or yellow onions
¼ cup bone broth
Sea salt and ground black pepper, to taste

Boil the potatoes until fork-tender.

Cook the lean beef in a nonstick pan.

Add the onions, bone broth, salt, and pepper. Simmer for 3 minutes.

Add the potato cubes and cook to combine.

Macros
Fat: 10 grams
Protein: 34 grams
Carbs: 52 grams

SALMON AND PINEAPPLE RICE BOWL

Lean, high-protein, bright feast-day meal.

Servings: 1

1 4-ounce wild salmon fillet
1 cup cooked white rice
½ cup pineapple chunks
1 tablespoon lime juice
Sea salt, to taste

Bake the salmon at 400°F (205°C) for 10 to 12 minutes with no added fat. Add the sea salt.

Combine the rice with the pineapple.

Drizzle the lime juice over the cooked salmon.

Macros
Fat: 8 grams
Protein: 32 grams
Carbs: 58 grams

CHICKEN APPLE RICE SKILLET

Naturally sweet, whole-food FEAST meal.

Servings: 1

1 6-ounce chicken breast, diced
1 medium apple, chopped
1 cup cooked white rice
Cinnamon
Pinch sea salt
1 teaspoon maple syrup (optional)

Cook the diced chicken in a nonstick skillet until cooked through and no pink juices run out.

Add the chopped apple and cook for 2 to 3 minutes.

Stir in the rice, cinnamon, and salt.

Add maple syrup, if desired.

Macros
Fat: 4 grams
Protein: 40 grams
Carbs: 55 grams

BANANA EGG-WHITE PANCAKES

Pure whole foods. Low fat. High protein. High carb.

Servings: 1

1 large ripe banana
4 egg whites
Cinnamon
2 tablespoons cassava flour OR 2 tablespoons white rice flour (optional, both low oxalate)
Pinch sea salt

Blend the banana, egg whites, cinnamon, and flour (if using) into a batter. Add sea salt.

Cook the batter into small pancakes in a lightly sprayed nonstick pan.

Flip when bubbles form.

Macros (with cassava or rice flour)
Fat: 2 grams
Protein: 31 grams
Carbs: 54 grams

AFTERWORD

Having completed the book, you may feel a bit overwhelmed by all the information I've presented, almost like you've been blasted by a firehose of ideas. Imagine your health as a bucket. When you're born into this world, your bucket is mostly empty. It's lightweight and easy to carry. As you continue through life, your bucket gets filled up with a poor diet, negative thoughts, toxins, and other lifestyle stress factors. As your bucket becomes fuller and heavier, you start to experience symptoms. You may not have thought of them this way, but symptoms are gifts from the body.[1] They signal that something is awry, and you need to take action. You wouldn't ignore the check-engine light in your car, right? The truth is that many people do ignore their symptoms, or they mask them with pills, supplements, or even elective surgery. You've been brainwashed to believe that symptoms and disease are evil, but the truth is, these are beautiful gifts from your innate intelligence. Let's pay attention to them. If your bucket continues to get full, eventually it overflows, leading to a serious problem. This book is intended to teach you how to empty your bucket by focusing on the underlying causes of your symptoms.

Take it one step at a time. If you need to, go back and review the chapters. Which solution did you feel like you could tackle first? If you can say, "Hey, I can do that!" then go ahead and try.

Success is never a straight line. There will be setbacks, but always remember to focus on the get-backs instead of the setbacks. When a rocket takes off with the goal of landing on the moon, it experiences several setbacks. It veers off course constantly. The GPS mechanism in place is continuously course correcting throughout its mission until the goal is achieved. You are the rocket in this scenario. Continue to course correct by revisiting the chapters in this book. You'll never fail if you never quit on yourself. Obstacles are learning opportunities.

As you embark on this new health journey, you'll quickly notice that new changes bring new problems. You may find your family members and friends are not supportive—they might even make fun of you. You may miss some of your favorite comfort foods that were loaded with sugar. When you stretch outside your comfort zone, it tends to suck. I've been there and continue to experience this suckiness. Here is my formula for success, which I hope you adopt: Suck, suck, SUCCESS! Embrace the suck, and keep pushing forward with the goal of beating yesterday.

I wrote this book to empower you to become a genius at mastering your good health. The four pillars in Keto Flex will move you from a path of building disease to a path of building vitality. You now have the keys to the perfect health kingdom. Apply what you've learned, and your future self will thank you for it.

I have so much gratitude for you. Always remember this: Your body was built to be self-healing. Don't let anyone convince you otherwise. My name is Ben, and I'm your friend. I love you.

Until next time . . .

APPENDIX A

Glossary of Most-Used Keto Terms

In this book, there may be words that are new to you. At first these terms can feel complicated, but as you learn to keto flex, you will see these terms often, so it's good to familiarize yourself with them.

Alternate-day fasting (ADF): Alternate-day fasting is a subtype of intermittent fasting and is defined as a continuous sequence of a fast day (100 percent energy restriction, zero calories) and a feed day (ad libitum food consumption). In the context of this book, we utilize this in back-to-back 24-hour periods.

Autophagy: A process by which a cell breaks down and destroys old, damaged, or abnormal proteins and other substances in its cytoplasm (the fluid inside a cell). The breakdown products are then recycled for important cell functions, especially during periods of fasting. This can happen after the 16 to 18 hours of fasting but can happen sooner or later depending on your metabolic health.

Basal metabolic rate (BMR): The rate at which the body uses energy while at rest to keep vital functions going, such as breathing and keeping warm. In short, this is the number of calories your body would burn if you sat on the couch all day. Overweight people who have calorically restricted typically have lower basal metabolic rates.

Blood sugar: The blood glucose level is the amount of glucose in the blood. Glucose is a sugar that comes from the foods we eat, and it's also formed and stored inside the body via liver and muscle cells. Healthy blood sugar should be between 70 and 90 mg/dL (milligrams per deciliter) when in a fasted state.

Breaking a fast: The term *breakfast* simply means you are "breaking your fast" from not eating food overnight. We also use this term to refer to a food or drink that raises blood sugar and starts the digestive system, thus turning off the healing benefits of being in a fasted state. In short, this means you have pulled yourself out of a fast and into a fed state.

Eating window: The period throughout your day when you are eating. You should eat all your meals and snacks within a particular window of time each day. This timeframe can vary according to the person's preference and the plan they choose to follow.

Fasting window: The period throughout your day when you are not eating or drinking beverages that raise glucose. Any food or drink that raises blood sugar and starts the digestive process will pull you out of your fasted window.

Fat adapted: Fat adaptation can occur to different degrees and across a spectrum dependent on the degree of carb restriction. This usually occurs when carbohydrates are restricted to under 50 total grams per day, over a period of seven days. You are fat adapted when you have shifted your body away from burning primarily sugar (glucose) to burning fat (ketones).

Keto adapted: Keto adaptation represents a more comprehensive reshaping of many physiologic systems, including how the body produces energy, regulates hormones, manages inflammation, and communicates hunger and satiety signals. Rather than simply burning fat, the body becomes more metabolically flexible and efficient at using ketones as a primary fuel source. Keto adaptation happens only when carbs are restricted to a point that induces sustained nutritional ketosis. This process takes longer than fat adaption. It is estimated to take 6 to 12 weeks.

Intermittent fasting: Going without food for 13 to 20 hours.

Insulin: A hormone made by the islet cells of the pancreas. Insulin controls the amount of sugar in the blood by moving it into the cells, where it can be used by the body for energy. Insulin is the primary fat-storage hormone.

Insulin resistance: Insulin resistance is when cells in your muscles, fat, and liver don't respond well to insulin and can't easily take up glucose from your blood. As a result, your pancreas makes more insulin to help glucose enter your cells. A more accurate term would be *hyperinsulinemia*. If not corrected, over time this can lead to prediabetes, and eventually diabetes.

Ketones: The signal that your liver is now burning energy from fat, not sugar. Ketones are a by-product of fat metabolism. The liver creates three different types of ketones: acetone, measured in the breath; acetoacetate, measured in the urine; and beta-hydroxybutyrate (BHB), measured in the blood. I suggest testing blood ketone measurements for BHB. The optimal ketone range is 0.8–3.0 mmol/L (millimoles per liter).

Ketosis: A metabolic process that happens when your body doesn't have enough carbohydrates to burn for energy. When you restrict carbohydrates in your diet, you lower the hormone insulin, which allows for fat burning. You can enter ketosis the preferred way, endogenously (from within) by burning fat for fuel, or exogenously (from outside) from exogenous ketones.

Keto flexing: Going in and out of ketosis after you've taught your body to be a fat burner. Some people call this carbohydrate cycling or keto cycling.

Metabolic flexibility: Being metabolically flexible enough to switch between burning sugar (glucose) and burning fat (ketones) without any problems.

Mitochondria: Mitochondria (*mitochondrion*, singular) are membrane-bound cell organelles that generate most of the chemical energy needed to power the cell's biochemical reactions. Chemical energy produced by the mitochondria is stored in a small molecule called adenosine triphosphate (ATP). Mitochondria contain their own small chromosomes. Mitochondria are also called the powerhouse of the cell.

mTOR: This stands for "mammalian target of rapamycin," a cellular-signaling pathway that gets triggered when amino acids and insulin levels within the cell increase. Usually this happens in the fed state. It stimulates anabolic growth and runs counter to autophagy, which is more catabolic in repair. Once stimulated, the mTOR pathway will promote cellular growth.

Stored sugar: The amount of glucose that is stored in tissues like the liver, fat, brain, muscle, and eyes.

Sugar burner: An energy system that burns fuel from the foods you eat. This energy system runs on the glucose created from food, primarily from carbohydrates.

Water fasting: A fast that involves drinking only water. This means a period (usually more than 16 hours) without food, only water.

APPENDIX B

Keto Flex Cooking and Food Lists

BEST WAYS TO COOK FOOD

- Heat lightly
- Steam
- Bake at 320°F or below
- Simmer
- Boil
- Poach
- Lightly grill (do not char)
- Sous vide
- Slow cook
- Pressure cook

WORST WAYS TO COOK FOOD

- Broil
- Barbecue
- Burn
- Blacken
- Char
- Deep-fry
- Microwave

AVOID THE FOLLOWING DIRTY-KETO FOODS

- Corn oil
- Soybean oil
- Fried foods
- Factory-chicken fat
- Sunflower oil
- Grain-fed beef
- Farmed fish
- Safflower oil

- Refined peanut oil
- Fish oil
- Canola oil (rapeseed oil in the UK)
- Cottonseed oil
- Margarine
- Legumes (including peanuts and chickpeas)
- Corn
- Raisins
- Dried fruit
- Jam
- Jelly
- Soy milk
- Diet drinks and soda
- Burned/blackened meat
- Spinach
- Almonds, almond flour, and almond milk
- Potato starch
- Powdered milk
- Pasteurized cow dairy
- Nightshades (tomatoes, potatoes, goji berries, peppers, eggplant)
- Soy
- Dairy replacer
- Condensed or evaporated milk
- Conventional ice cream
- Wheat and grains
- Corn
- Millet
- Cornstarch
- Garbanzo flour

APPROVED OILS AND FATS

- Unrefined coconut oil
- Grass-fed beef tallow
- Pastured egg yolks
- Duck fat
- Grass-fed animal fat and marrow
- Avocado oil
- Grass-fed butter
- Sunflower lecithin
- Grass-fed ghee
- Cacao butter
- Bulletproof Brain Octane MCT Oil
- Dark chocolate

- Palm oil
- Palm kernel oil
- Extra-virgin olive oil
- Pastured bacon fat
- MCT oil
- MCT powder

APPROVED NUTS, SEEDS, AND LEGUMES

- Coconut
- Coconut flour
- Cashews
- Chestnuts
- Hazelnuts
- Macadamia
- Pili nuts
- Pecans
- Walnuts
- Sunflower seeds
- Cashew flour
- Pecan flour
- Walnut meal/flour
- Nut butters (except peanut and almond)
- Sunflower seed butter
- Pine nuts

APPROVED PROTEINS

- Grass-fed beef and lamb
- Pastured eggs and gelatin
- Colostrum
- Collagen protein
- Beef gelatin
- Marine collagen
- Wild anchovies
- Wild haddock
- Wild sardines
- Wild sockeye salmon
- Wild summer flounder
- Wild trout
- Grass-fed whey
- Pastured pork
- Pastured duck and goose
- Hemp protein
- Bone broth
- Organic, free-range poultry

APPROVED FRUIT AND CARBOHYDRATES FOR KETO FLEX DAYS

- Avocado
- Grapes
- Guava
- Blackberries
- Mango
- Coconut
- Melons
- Cranberries
- Papaya
- Lemon
- Passion fruit
- Lime
- Plantain
- Raspberries
- Watermelon
- Blueberries
- Asparagus
- Pineapple
- Bok choy
- Strawberries
- Broccoli
- Tangerine
- Brussels sprouts
- Grapefruit
- Cauliflower
- Pomegranate
- Celery
- Apple
- Cucumber
- Apricot
- Fennel
- Cherries
- Olives
- Figs
- Kiwi
- Cooked collards
- Lychee
- Cabbage
- Nectarine
- Lettuce
- Orange
- Radishes
- Peach
- Pears
- Summer squash
- Plums
- Zucchini
- Bananas
- Dates
- Cilantro
- Arrowroot
- Resistant-starch powder
- Pumpkin
- Plantain flour

- Butternut squash
- Black rice
- Sweet potato
- Wild rice
- Yam
- Brown rice
- Carrot
- Artichokes
- White rice
- Zucchini
- Cassava
- Winter squash
- Taro
- Green beans
- Tapioca flour/starch
- Green onion
- Leeks
- Approved Dairy
- Colostrum
- Grass-fed ghee or butter
- Grass-fed cream
- Grass-fed sheep's yogurt
- Full-fat, raw A2 milk or yogurt
- Grass-fed cow cheese
- Raw sheep/goat cheese
- Raw kefir (cow, sheep, goat)
- Approved Keto Sweeteners
- Erythritol
- Pure stevia
- Monk fruit
- Xylitol
- Swerve
- Keto Flex Day Sweeteners
- D-ribose
- Non-GMO dextrose
- Glucose
- Raw honey
- Maple syrup
- Coconut sugar
- Blackstrap molasses

NONAPPROVED SWEETENERS

- Sorbitol
- Acesulfame potassium
- Mannitol
- Aspartame
- Sucralose
- Saccharin

APPROVED BEVERAGES

- Unsweetened tea
- Zevia soda
- Swoon
- Organic coffee
- E-lyte water
- Electrolyte powders
- Spring water
- Hydrogen water
- Coconut milk
- Cashew milk
- Hazelnut milk
- Macadamia nut milk

APPROVED ON-THE-GO KETO FOODS

- Canned sardines
- Oysters
- Sockeye salmon
- Mackerel
- Anchovies
- Raw macadamia nuts
- Roasted nori seaweed crackers
- Hard-boiled or deviled eggs
- Raw coconut butter
- Guacamole with EPIC bars or PaleoValley beef sticks
- Pastured pork rinds
- Bacon "chips"
- Avocados
- Homemade fat bombs
- Grass-fed cheese/yogurt
- Sugar-free jerky
- High-fat smoothies and puddings
- Homemade unsweetened ice pops
- Plant-based pea-protein powder
- Bulletproof and EPIC Bars
- PaleoValley Beef Sticks

ENDNOTES

Chapter 1

1. "How Many Cells Are in Your Body? Probably More Than You Think!" Eppendorf, n.d., https://www.eppendorf.com/us-en/beyond-science/health-medicine/how-many-cells-are-in-your-body-probably-more-than-you-think.

2. John E. Hall, *Guyton and Hall Textbook of Medical Physiology*, 12th ed. (Saunders/Elsevier, 2011), #.

3. H. Stephen Stoker, *General, Organic, and Biological Chemistry*, 4th ed. (Cengage-Learning, 2006); Ivan G. Darvey, "How Does the Ratio of ATP Yield from the Complete Oxidation of Palmitic Acid to that of Glucose Compare with the Relative Energy Contents of Fat and Carbohydrate?" *Biochemical Education* 26, no. 1 (January 1998), 22–3, https://doi.org/10.1016/S0307-4412(97)00046-0; Viorica Meltzer, Elena Pincu, and Gabriela Cristescu, "Heat of Combustion of Some Saturated Dicarboxylic Acids from Group Contributions," *Analele Universității din București—Chimie* 16 (new series), no. 1 (2007): 21–4, https://www.researchgate.net/publication/26609620_HEAT_OF_COMBUSTION_OF_SOME_SATURATED_DICARBOXYLIC_ACIDS_FROM_GROUP_CONTRIBUTIONS; Lodish et al., *Molecular Cell Biology*, 4th ed. (New York: W. H. Freeman, 1999); Kanit Krisnangkura, "Estimation of Heat of Combustion of Triglycerides and Fatty Acid Methyl Esters," *Journal of the American Oil Chemists Society* 68, no. 1 (January 1991): 56–8, https://doi.org/10.1007/BF02660311.

4. Labrie et al., "Effect of Intravaginal DHEA on Serum DHEA and Eleven of Its Metabolites in Postmenopausal Women," *The Journal of Steroid Biochemistry and Molecular Biology* 111, no. 3-5 (September 2008): 178–94, https://doi.org/10.1016/j.jsbmb.2008.06.003.; Henry G. Burger, "Androgen Production in Women," *Fertility and Sterility* 77, suppl 4 (April 2002): 3–5, https://www.fertstert.org/article/S0015-0282(02)02985-0/fulltext.

5. Brann et al., "Neurotrophic and Neuroprotective Actions of Estrogen: Basic Mechanisms and Clinical Implications," *Steroids* 72, no. 5 (May 2007): 381–405, https://doi.org/10.1016/j.steroids.2007.02.003.

6. Marie-Pierre St.-Onge, "The Role of Sleep Duration in the Regulation of Energy Balance: Effects on Energy Intakes and Expenditure," *Journal of Clinical Sleep Medicine* 9, no. 1 (January 15, 2013): 73–80, https://doi.org/10.5664/jcsm.2348.

Chapter 2

1. "Excerpts from the Writings of Paramahansa Yogananda: From the Talk 'Healing by God's Unlimited Power,'" Self-Realization Fellowship, https://yogananda.org/health-and-healing.

2. Bhaddāli Sutta (MN 65), *Majjhima Nikāya*, trans. Bhikkhu Ñānamoli and Bhikkhu Bodhi, in *The Middle Length Discourses of the Buddha* (Boston: Wisdom Publications, 1995).

3. Plutarch, *Moralia*, trans. Frank Cole Babbitt et al., Loeb Classical Library (Cambridge, MA: Harvard University Press, 1927–2004).

4. Paracelsus, *Selected Writings*, trans. Norbert Guterman (Princeton, NJ: Princeton University Press, 1951).

5. Benjami Franklin, *The Autobiography and Other Writings* (New York: Oxford University Press, 2008).

6. Herbert M. Shelton, *Fasting Can Save Your Life* (San Antonio, TX: Shelton's Health School, 1954).

7. Wilkinson et al., "Ten-Hour Time-Restricted Eating Reduces Weight, Blood Pressure, and Atherogenic Lipids in Patients with Metabolic Syndrome," *Cell Metabolism* 31, no. 1 (January 2020): 92–104.e5, https://doi.org/10.1016/j.cmet.2019.11.004.

8. Sutton et al., "Early Time-Restricted Feeding Improves Insulin Sensitivity, Blood Pressure, and Oxidative Stress Even Without Weight Loss in Men with Prediabetes," *Cell Metabolism* 27, no. 6 (June 2018): 1212–21.e3, https://doi.org/10.1016/j.cmet.2018.04.010.

9. "More Than 100 Million Americans Have High Blood Pressure, AHA Says," American Heart Association, January 31, 2018, https://www.heart.org/en/news/2018/07/18/more-than-100-million-americans-have-high-blood-pressure-aha-says.

10. Anne Trafton, "Fasting Boosts Stem Cells' Regenerative Capacity." MIT News, Massachusetts Institute of Technology, June 7, 2018, https://news.mit.edu/2018/fasting-boosts-stem-cells-regenerativecapacit.

11. Godínez-Victoria et al., "Intermittent Fasting Promotes Bacterial Clearance and Intestinal IgA Production in Salmonella Typhimurium-Infected Mice," *Scandinavian Journal of Immunology* 79, no. 5 (April 20, 2014): 315–24, https://doi.org/10.1111/sji.12163; Guolin et al, "Intermittent Fasting Promotes White Adipose Browning and Decreases Obesity by Shaping the Gut Microbiota," *Cell Metabolism* 26, no. 4 (November 2017): 672-685.e4, https://www.cell.com/action/showMethods?pii=S1550-4131%2817%2930504-1; Noboru Mizushima and Tamotsu Yoshimori, "Autophagy in Diabetes: β-Cell Dysfunction, Insulin Resistance, and Complications," *Annual Review of Nutrition*, vol. 35 (2015): 51–74, https://www.ncbi.nlm.nih.gov/pmc/articles/PMC6924600/.

12. Lucy Danziger, "Surprising Ways to Lower Your Cancer Risk at Any Age From a Doctor." The Beet, June 21, 2021, https://thebeet.com/surprising-ways-to-lower-your-cancer-risk-at-any-age-from-a-doctor; University of California—San Diego, "When—Not What—Obese Mice Ate Reduced Breast Cancer Risk," *ScienceDaily*, January 27, 2021, https://www.sciencedaily.com/releases/2021/01/210125191806.htm.

13. Jason Fung, "How to Fix Your Broken Metabolism by Doing the Exact Opposite," The Fasting Method, May 12, 2016, https://www.thefastingmethod.com/how-to-fix-your-broken-metabolism-by-doing-the-exact-opposite/.

Chapter 3

1. Ge et al., "Comparison of Dietary Macronutrient Patterns of 14 Popular Named Dietary Programmes for Weight and Cardiovascular Risk Factor Reduction in Adults: Systematic Review and Network Meta-Analysis of Randomised Trials," *BMJ* 369, no. 8240 (April 1, 2020): m696, https://doi.org/10.1136/bmj.m696.

2. Kevin D. Hall and Scott Kahan, "Maintenance of Lost Weight and Long-Term Management of Obesity," *Medical Clinics of North America* 102, no. 1 (January 2018): 183–197, https://doi.org/10.1016/j.mcna.2017.08.012.

3. P. D. MacLean, *The Triune Brain in Evolution: Role in Paleocerebral Functions* (New York: Plenum Press, 1990).

4. Debras et al., "Artificial Sweeteners and Cancer Risk: Results from the NutriNet-Santé Population-Based Cohort Study," *PLOS Medicine* 19, no. 3 (2022): e1003950, https://doi.org/10.1371/journal.pmed.1003950.

5. Debras et al., "Artificial Sweeteners and Risk of Cardiovascular Diseases: Results from the Prospective NutriNet-Santé Cohort," *BMJ* 378, no. 8351 (September 7, 2022), https://doi.org/10.1136/bmj-2022-071204; Lindseth et al., "Neurobehavioral Effects of Aspartame Consumption," *Research in Nursing and Health* 37, no. 3 (June 2014): 185–93, https://doi.org/10.1002/nur.21595.

6. Stacy Malkan, "Aspartame: Decades of Science Point to Health Risks," U.S. Right to Know, March 27, 2025, https://usrtk.org/sweeteners/aspartame_health_risks/.

7. Jensen et al., "Effects of Ketone Bodies on Brain Metabolism and Function in Neurodegenerative Diseases," *International Journal of Molecular Sciences* 21, no. 22 (November 20, 2020): 8767, http://doi.org10.3390/ijms21228767.

8. Mavropoulos et al., "The Effects of a Low-Carbohydrate, Ketogenic Diet on the Polycystic Ovary Syndrome: A Pilot Study," *Nutrition and Metabolism (London)* 2 (December 16, 2005): 35, https://doi.org/10.1186/1743-7075-2-35.

9. Maalouf et al., "Ketones Inhibit Mitochondrial Production of Reactive Oxygen Species Production Following Glutamate Excitotoxicity by Increasing NADH Oxidation." *Neuroscience* 145, no. 1 (January 18, 2007): 256–64, https://doi.org/10.1016/j.neuroscience.2006.11.065.

10. Yurista et al., "Therapeutic Potential of Ketone Bodies for Patients with Cardiovascular Disease: *JACC* State-of-the-Art Review," *JACC* 77, no. 13 (April 2021): 1660–9, https://doi.org/10.1016/j.jacc.2020.12.065.

11. Newman et al., "Ketogenic Diet Reduces Midlife Mortality and Improves Memory in Aging Mice," *Cell Metabolism* 26, no. 3 (September 5, 2017): 547–57, https://doi.org/10.1016/j.cmet.2017.08.004.

12. Shimazu et al., "Suppression of Oxidative Stress by β-Hydroxybutyrate, an Endogenous Histone Deacetylase Inhibitor," *Science* 339, no. 6116 (January 11, 2013): 211–4, https://doi.org/10.1126/science.1227166.

13. Roberts et al., "A Ketogenic Diet Extends Longevity and Healthspan in Adult Mice," *Cell Metabolism* 26, no. 3 (September 5, 2017): 539–546, https://doi.org/10.1016/j.cmet.2017.08.005.

14. Adam L. Hartman and Jong M. Rho, "The New Ketone Alphabet Soup: BHB, HCA, and HDAC," *American Epilepsy Society* 14, no. 6 (November 1, 2014), https://doi.org/10.5698/1535-7597-14.6.355.

Chapter 4

1. Nader Rahmi and Sonu Gupta, "Biochemistry, Ketogenesis. [Updated December 1, 2025]." *StatPearls* Internet (Treasure Island, FL: StatPearls, 2025), www.ncbi.nlm.nih.gov/books/NBK493179/.

2. G. Guelpa and A. Marie, "La Lutte Contre L'épilepsie Par La Désintoxication Et Par La Rééducation Alimentaire," *Revue de Thérapeutique Médico-Chirurgicale* 78 (1911): 8–13.

3. "Obesity and Overweight," National Center for Health Statistics, reviewed January 27, 2026, https://www.cdc.gov/nchs/fastats/obesity-overweight.htm.

4. John Anderer, "Food Fads: The Average Adult Will Try 126 Different Diets During Their Life!" StudyFinds, updated May 18, 2022, https://www.studyfinds.org/food-fads-the-average-adult-will-try-126different-diets-during-their-life/.

5. Mustieles et al., "Bisphenol A and Its Analogues in Environmental Health: Emerging Tools for Risk Assessment." *International Journal of Molecular Sciences*, vol. 21, no. 24 (2020), https://doi.org/10.1016/j.envint.2020.105811.

6. Philip Barter, "The Role of HDL-Cholesterol in Preventing Atherosclerotic Disease," *European Heart Journal Supplements* 7, suppl_F (July 2005): F4–8, https://doi.org/10.1093/eurheartj/sui036; Linton et al., "HDL Function and Atherosclerosis: Reactive Dicarbonyls as Promising Targets of Therapy," *Circulation Research* 132, no. 11 (May 26, 2023): 1521–45, https://doi.org/10.1161/CIRCRESAHA.123.321563.

7. David Tak Wai Lui and Kathryn Choon Beng Tan, "High-Density Lipoprotein in Diabetes: Structural and Functional Relevance," *Journal of Diabetes Investigation* 15, no. 7 (February 28, 2024): 805–16, https://doi.org/10.1111/jdi.14172; Rohatgi et al., "HDL in the 21st Century: A Multifunctional Roadmap for Future HDL Research," *Circulation* 143, no. 23 (June 8, 2021): 2293–309, https://doi.org/10.1161/CIRCULATIONAHA.120.044221; Bonacina et al., "HDL in Immune-Inflammatory Responses: Implications Beyond Cardiovascular Diseases," *Cells* 10, no. 5 (April 29, 2021): 1061, https://doi.org/10.3390/cells10051061.

Chapter 5

1. Staff Writer, "Close to Half of U.S. Population Projected to Have Obesity by 2030," press release, Harvard T.H. Chan School of Public Health, December 18, 2019, https://hsph.harvard.edu/news/half-of-us-to-have-obesity-by-2030.

2. Ryan Rodal, "Ketosis: Keto Electrolytes Tips and Concerns." *Ketone IQ Blog*, updated November 15, 2019, https://hvmn.com/blogs/blog/ketosis-keto-electrolytes-tips-and-concerns.

3. Michael Lieberman and Allan D. Marks, *Marks' Basic Medical Biochemistry: A Clinical Approach*, 3rd ed. (Philadelphia, PA: Lippincott, Williams and Wilkins, 2009), 653.

4. Brian Scott Peskin with Stephen Cavallino, *The 24-Hour Diet: The No-Denial Strategy of Fabulous Food to Make You Lean-for-Life* (Pinnacle Press, 2007).

5. Paleo Leaper, "Bitterness: The Taste We Bred Out of Modern Food and How to Get It Back," PaleoLeap, last modified February 22, 2023, https://paleoleap.com/bitterness-modern-food.

Chapter 6

1. Hartman et al., "Augmented Growth Hormone (GH) Secretory Burst Frequency and Amplitude Mediate Enhanced GH Secretion During a Two-Day Fast in Normal Men," *Journal of Clinical Endocrinology and Metabolism* 74, no. 4 (April 1, 1992): 757–765, https://doi.org/10.1210/jcem.74.4.1548337.

2. Jamshed et al., "Effectiveness of Early Time-Restricted Eating for Weight Loss, Fat Loss, and Cardiometabolic Health in Adults with Obesity: A Randomized Clinical Trial," *JAMA Internal Medicine* 182, no. 9 (September 1, 2022): 953–962. https://doi.org/10.1001/jamainternmed.2022.3050.

Chapter 7

1. Shen et al., "Potential Immunoregulatory Mechanism of Plant Saponins: A Review," *Molecules* 29, no. 1 (2024): 113, https://doi.org/10.3390/molecules29010113.

2. Caleb J. Kelly, "A Controlled Trial of Reduced Meal Frequency Without Caloric Restriction in Healthy, Normal-Weight, Middle-Aged Adults," *American Journal of Clinical Nutrition* 86, no. 4 (October 2007):1254–1255. https://ajcn.nutrition.org/article/S0002-9165(23)13500-3/fulltext; Ellenbroek et al., "Long-Term Ketogenic Diet Causes Glucose Intolerance and Reduced β- and α-Cell Mass but No Weight Loss in Mice," *American Journal of Physiology-Endocrinology and Metabolism* 306, no. 5 (January 7, 2014): E552–E558, https://journals.physiology.org/doi/full/10.1152/ajpendo.00453.2013.

3. Brad Pilon, *Eat Stop Eat: Intermittent Fasting for Health and Weight Loss* (Independently published, 2007).

Chapter 8

1. Françoise Guéraud, "4-Hydroxynonenal Metabolites and Adducts in Pre-Carcinogenic Conditions and Cancer," *Free Radical Biology and Medicine* 111 (October 2017): 196–208. https://doi.org/10.1016/j.freeradbiomed.2016.12.025.

Chapter 9

1. Ben Azadi, host, *Metabolic Freedom*, episode 102, "Why You're Not Losing Fat (Even If You're Doing Everything Right) – Game-Changing Fixes with Dr. Stephanie Estima," August 6, 2025.

2. Thompson et al., "Dietary Prebiotics and Bioactive Milk Fractions Improve NREM Sleep, Enhance REM Sleep Rebound and Attenuate the Stress-Induced Decrease in Diurnal Temperature and Gut Microbial Alpha Diversity," *Frontiers in Behavioral Neuroscience* 10 (2017): 240, https://doi.org/10.3389/fnbeh.2016.00240.

3. Najlaa M. Al-Mana and M. Denise Robertson, "Acute Effect of Resistant Starch on Food Intake, Appetite and Satiety in Overweight/Obese Males," *Nutrients* 10, no. 12 (2018): 1993, https://doi.org/10.3390/nu10121993.

4. Gentile et al., "Resistant Starch and Protein Intake Enhances Fat Oxidation and Feelings of Fullness in Lean and Overweight/Obese Women," *Nutrition Journal* 14 (October 29, 2015):113, https://doi.org/10.1186/s12937-015-0104-2.

Chapter 10

1. Ryan Rodal, "Ketosis: Keto Electrolytes Tips and Concerns," *Ketone-IQ Blog*, updated November 15, 2019, https://ketone.com/blogs/blog/ketosis-keto-electrolytes-tips-and-concerns.

2. Nicole M. Avena, Pedro Rada, and Bartley G. Hoebel, "Evidence for Sugar Addiction: Behavioral and Neurochemical Effects of Intermittent, Excessive Sugar Intake," *Neuroscience & Biobehavioral Reviews* 32, no. 1 (2008): 20–39. https://www.sciencedirect.com/science/article/abs/pii/S0149763407000589.

3. Nunes Santiago et al., "Oral Glutamine Is Superior than Oral Glucose to Promote Glycemia Recovery in Mice Submitted to Insulin-Induced Hypoglycemia," *International Journal of Endocrinology* 2013 (August 24, 2013): 841514, https://doi.org/10.1155/2013/841514.

4. Monica Reinagel, "Getting More Sleep Can Reduce Food Cravings," *Scientific American*, October 22, 2019, https://www.scientificamerican.com/article/getting-more-sleep-can-reduce-food-cravings/.

5. Desrochers et al., "Metabolism of R- and S-1,3-Butanediol in Perfused Livers from Meal-Fed and Starved Rats," *Biochemical Journal* 285, part II (July 15, 1992): 647–653. https://pubmed.ncbi.nlm.nih.gov/1637355.

6. Harvie et al., "The Effect of Intermittent Energy and Carbohydrate Restriction v. Daily Energy Restriction on Weight Loss and Metabolic Disease Risk Markers in Overweight Women," *British Journal of Nutrition* 110, no. 8 (October 2013): 1534–47, https://doi.org/10.1017/S0007114513000792.

7. Scott et al., "The Effect of 1,3-Butanediol and Carbohydrate Supplementation on Running Performance," *Journal of Science and Medicine in Sport* 22, no. 6 (June 2019): 702–706. 10.1016/j.jsams.2018.11.027; Shaw et al., "The Effect of 1,3-Butanediol on Cycling Time-Trial Performance," *International Journal of Sport Nutrition and Exercise Metabolism* 29, no. 5 (2019): 466–473. 10.1123/ijsnem.2018-0284.

8. Teri B. O'Neal and Euil E. Luther, "Dawn Phenomenon [Updated May 16, 2023]." In: *StatPearls* Internet (Treasure Island, FL: StatPearls, 2023), https://www.ncbi.nlm.nih.gov/sites/books/NBK430893/.

9. Li et al., "The Dawn Phenomenon Across the Glycemic Continuum: Implications for Defining Dysglycemia," *Diabetes Research and Clinical Practice* 166 (August 2020): 108308, https://doi.org/10.1016/j.diabres.2020.108308.

10. Li et al., "The Dawn Phenomenon Across the Glycemic Continuum."

11. Katherine Harmon, "How Slight Sleep Deprivation Could Add Extra Pounds," Scientific American, October 24, 2012, https://www.scientificamerican.com/article/sleep-deprivation-obesity/.

12. Vandenberghe et al., "Caffeine Intake Increases Plasma Ketones: An Acute Metabolic Study in Humans," *Canadian Journal of Physiology and Pharmacology* 95, no. 4 (April 2017): 455–58, https://doi.org/10.1139/cjpp-2016-0338.

13. Rejane Mattar, Daniel Ferraz de Campos Mazo, and Flair Jose Carrilho, "Lactose Intolerance: Diagnosis, Genetic, and Clinical Factors," *Clinical and Experimental Gastroenterology* 5 (2012): 113–21, https://doi.org/10.2147/ceg.s32368.

14. Op den Kamp-Bruls et al., "Carnitine Supplementation Improves Insulin Sensitivity and Skeletal Muscle Acetylcarnitine Formation in Patients with Type 2 Diabetes," *Diabetes, Obesity and Metabolism* 27, no. 5 (May 2025): 2864–2877, https://doi.org/10.1111/dom.16298.

INDEX

C

G

H

O

P

S

ACKNOWLEDGMENTS

Writing a book is an act of faith—and faith, as I have come to understand it, is the ability to see the invisible, believe in the incredible, and achieve what the masses think is impossible. Nowhere is this definition more alive than in the arena of health and healing. The human body's capacity to restore, regenerate, and renew itself is one of the greatest invisible forces on earth. Most people never witness it—not because it isn't real, but because they stopped believing before the miracle had a chance to arrive.

Keto Flex was not born in a laboratory or a library. It was born in the trenches of real transformation, forged through thousands of conversations with real people who were struggling, searching, and ultimately succeeding against odds that the mainstream medical world had already written off.

Since 2008, I have had the profound privilege of working alongside students and clients from every walk of life. They came to me exhausted, frustrated, and often told by the system that their suffering was simply the price of getting older. They refused to accept that answer—and because of their faith, neither did I. They chose to see what others couldn't. They chose to believe what others wouldn't. And in doing so, they achieved what the masses called impossible.

This book belongs to them.

To every student who has trusted me with their health journey over the past sixteen-plus years: You are the true authors of this work. Your willingness to show up, embrace the hard things, and hold on to belief when results felt distant has shaped every principle contained in these pages. I have learned far more from you than you will ever know.

It is a rare and humbling thing to witness a human being reclaim their life. I have been fortunate enough to witness it thousands of times—and every single time, faith was the ingredient that made the difference. Not certainty. Not perfection. Faith.

Thank you for being my greatest teachers. Thank you for showing me, and the world, what becomes possible when you refuse to stop believing.

ABOUT THE AUTHOR

Ben Azadi, FDN-P, is the *New York Times* best-selling author of *Metabolic Freedom*, an international keynote speaker, and a metabolic health expert with over 17 years of experience helping thousands reclaim their health. A recognized leader in the alternative health field, Ben is a pioneer in the keto and fasting movement, teaching the principles of a keto lifestyle, fasting, detox, hormone balance, and overall metabolic function.

His popular YouTube channel, where he shares the latest science-backed tools and techniques for resetting metabolism, has garnered over 100 million views. Ben is also the host of the *Metabolic Freedom* podcast, a top-15 podcast with more than 85 million downloads and more than 1300 episodes. The podcast was honored as Keto Podcast of the Year (2022) by the Metabolic Health Summit.

Ben's work has been featured in major publications such as *Forbes*, *LA Weekly*, *Disrupt* magazine, *Men's Health*, *Psychology Today*, *New York Times Magazine*, and *LA Entertainment Weekly*. He also appeared in the groundbreaking documentary *Biohack Yourself* on Amazon Prime.

To learn more about Ben Azadi and his work, visit **benazadi.com**.

Hay House Titles of Related Interest

YOU CAN HEAL YOUR LIFE, the movie,
starring Louise Hay & Friends
(available as an online streaming video)
www.hayhouse.com/louise-movie

THE SHIFT, the movie,
starring Dr. Wayne W. Dyer
(available as an online streaming video)
www.hayhouse.com/the-shift-movie

***

BOUNDLESS KITCHEN: Biohack Your Body & Boost Your Brain with Healthy Recipes You Actually Want to Eat, by Ben Greenfield

FAST LIKE A GIRL: A Woman's Guide to Using the Healing Power of Fasting to Burn Fat, Boost Energy, and Balance Hormones, by Dr. Mindy Pelz

LIFE-CHANGING FOODS EXPANDED EDITION: Save Yourself & Your Loved Ones with Fruits, Leafy Greens, Herbs, Wild Foods & Vegetables, by Anthony William

POWERED BY PLANTS: Nutrient-Loaded 30-Minute Meals to Help You Thrive, by Ocean Robbins and Nichole Dandrea-Russert, MS, RDN

All of the above are available at your local bookstore, or may be ordered by contacting Hay House (see next page).

***

We hope you enjoyed this Hay House book. If you'd like to receive our online catalog featuring additional information on Hay House books and products, or if you'd like to find out more about the Hay Foundation, please contact:

Hay House LLC, P.O. Box 5100, Carlsbad, CA 92018-5100
(760) 431-7695 or (800) 654-5126
www.hayhouse.com® • www.hayfoundation.org

Published in Australia by:
Hay House Australia Publishing Pty Ltd
18/36 Ralph St., Alexandria NSW 2015
Phone: +61 (02) 9669 4299
www.hayhouse.com.au

Published in the United Kingdom by:
Hay House UK Ltd
1st Floor, Crawford Corner,
91–93 Baker Street, London W1U 6QQ
Phone: +44 (0)20 3927 7290
www.hayhouse.co.uk

Published in India by:
Hay House Publishers (India) Pvt Ltd
Muskaan Complex, Plot No. 3,
B-2, Vasant Kunj, New Delhi 110 070
Phone: +91 11 41761620
www.hayhouse.co.in
